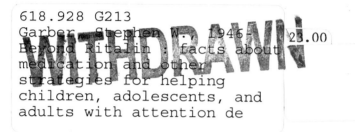
DATE DUE		
OCT 27	APR 2 5 1999	
FEB 13 1997		
MAR 3 1 1997	JUN 2 4 1998	
JUN 18 1997	DEC 1 2 1999	
7/17/97	DEC 2 0 1999	
JUL 1 7 1997	SEP 1 8 2001	
AUG 6 1997	3.24.03	
OCT 8 1997	NOV 1 1 2005	
OCT 3 0 1998	MAY 1 7 2006	
NOV 1 6 1998		
DEC 3 1998		
MAR 1 9 1999		

201-9500   PRINTED IN U.S.A.

Also by Stephen W. Garber, Ph.D.,
Marianne Daniels Garber, Ph.D., and
Robyn Freedman Spizman:

*IS YOUR CHILD HYPERACTIVE? INATTENTIVE? IMPULSIVE? DISTRACTIBLE?
HELPING THE ADD/HYPERACTIVE CHILD*

*MONSTERS UNDER THE BED AND OTHER CHILDHOOD FEARS:
HELPING YOUR CHILD OVERCOME ANXIETIES, FEARS AND PHOBIAS*

*GOOD BEHAVIOR: OVER 1,200 SOLUTIONS TO YOUR CHILD'S PROBLEMS FROM
BIRTH TO AGE TWELVE*

BEYOND RITALIN

FACTS ABOUT MEDICATION AND OTHER
STRATEGIES FOR HELPING
CHILDREN, ADOLESCENTS,
AND ADULTS WITH
ATTENTION DEFICIT DISORDERS

BEYOND RITALIN

Facts About Medication and
Other Strategies for Helping
Children, Adolescents,
and Adults with
Attention Deficit Disorders

Stephen W. Garber, Ph.D.

Marianne Daniels Garber, Ph.D.

Robyn Freedman Spizman

VILLARD
NEW YORK

**THIS BOOK IS NOT IN ANY WAY
SPONSORED BY, CONNECTED TO, OR ASSOCIATED WITH
THE MANUFACTURERS OF RITALIN.**

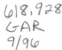

Copyright © 1996 by Marianne Garber, Ph.D., Stephen W. Garber, Ph.D.,
and Robyn Freedman Spizman

Grateful acknowledgment is made to American Psychiatric Association for
permission to reprint "Diagnostic Criteria for Attention-Deficit/Hyperactivity
Disorder" from American Psychiatric Association: *Diagnostic and Statistical
Manual of Mental Disorders, Fourth Edition* (Washington, D.C.: American
Psychiatric Association, 1994). Reprinted by permission.

LIBRARY OF CONGRESS CATALOGING-IN-PUBLICATION DATA IS AVAILABLE

ISBN 0-679-45018-1

Printed in the United States of America on acid-free paper

9 8 7 6 5 4 3 2

First Edition

The names of the individuals involved in examples and case histories used in this book have been changed. We have randomly interchanged the pronouns used in the book. Although ADHD still appears to afflict more males than females, most often examples reflect experiences that could be those of either sex. When reading the information, feel free to think of the children, adolescents, and adults you know best.

In addition, please note that the terms *attention deficit hyperactivity disorder* (ADHD) and *attention deficit disorder* (ADD) are labels used interchangeably to designate the same constellation of symptoms. Although ADD is the more popularly recognized term, ADHD is the name given to the disorder by the American Psychiatric Association in its *Diagnostic and Statistical Manual of Mental Disorders,* Fourth Edition (*DSM-IV*). In *Beyond Ritalin* we most often use the technically correct term ADHD to denote all forms of attention deficit disorders including those with and without hyperactivity.

FOREWORD

For the past twenty years we have been working with children and adolescents who suffer from the complex problem now called attention deficit hyperactivity disorder (ADHD). In our personal lives, we have grappled with the issues surrounding ADHD, so we know firsthand how difficult and troubling the problems associated with this disorder can be.

We have written *Beyond Ritalin* because we now know that there is so much that can and must be done, far beyond medication alone, to help those who suffer from ADHD. In the beginning we thought we could help these youngsters without medication, using the behavioral techniques that had worked well for so many others with behavior problems at home and school. Along the way, though, we discovered that for many children medication made a significant difference, permitting the youngsters to sit longer, pay attention better, control impulsiveness, and be receptive to other kinds of therapy and instruction they needed.

Medication for ADHD remains a controversial, often misunderstood issue, so we must be clear: Medication does not cure ADHD; it doesn't teach the child how to follow directions in school, sit and do homework, make and keep friends, or be less forgetful. *Beyond Ritalin* presents a close look, based on current research, at what medication can and cannot do for those with ADHD.

While ADHD has been traditionally considered a childhood problem, *Beyond Ritalin* is not written just about children and parents. As we followed the youngsters we worked with through the years, we saw that many of them grew into young men and women still dealing with many aspects of the disorder. In addition, many of their parents recognized in themselves the symptoms that define this disorder. However, other adults have also begun to ask if they might have ADHD. For the first time they were able to give a name to the troubling characteristics that had wreaked havoc with their lives.

It became clear to us, as it has to so many other professionals, that ADHD is not simply a childhood problem. *Beyond Ritalin* is written to help individuals of all ages, and the people who care about them, understand what they can and must do to help themselves.

In the 1980s, national attention came to ADHD and the medication most prescribed for it, Ritalin. The glare of the spotlight brought reasonable concern and fear. Were too many children being placed on medication? Was ADHD a scapegoat for discipline problems in the schools? In the midst of controversy, however, other important questions were lost. The questions each parent and individual must ask are: Do I have a correct diagnosis of ADHD? What kind of medication might be helpful? What else can and should I do to help myself or my child deal with this problem? At the risk of sounding trite, **"To take Ritalin or not to take Ritalin"** is not the only issue.

Perhaps you picked up this book because you are facing the decision of what to do about ADHD for yourself or your child. Or you may have already chosen to use medication, but don't have a clear understanding about what it does. You may have elected not to use medication and want to know what other kinds of treatment are available. We have written *Beyond Ritalin* to answer each of your concerns and serve as a guide to coping with and overcoming each troubling aspect of this disorder.

On a daily basis we see people whose quality of life has been affected by ADHD. We have met individuals who have and haven't been helped by various medications, and those who have found other ways to cope with this problem. We dedicate this book to all of these people, who have the courage to ask the really hard questions, to challenge professionals to find additional answers, and to be willing to search for solutions beyond Ritalin.

ACKNOWLEDGMENTS

As with every manuscript and project—in fact, as with everything we do—there are many people to whom we owe thanks. First, we thank our families for giving us the support and encouragement to accomplish our goals: Robyn's husband Willy; the Garber children: Amy, Adam, Arielle, and Aubrey; the Spizman children: Justin and Ali; our parents: Al and Gerry Garber, Rose Daniels and the late Dan Daniels, Phyllis and Jack Freedman; Gus Spizman and the late Regina Spizman; our friends Doris Dozier and Bettye Storne, without whom no job would be completed.

We are indebted to Robyn Liebman for the countless hours she spent in research for us; Dr. Lyndon Waugh; Dr. Noelle Gregg; Betsy Primm; Dr. Mark McElhaney; Dr. Rick Carpenter; the late Dr. Randy Gerson and Dr. Kathleen O'Toole, who read the manuscript and made suggestions; and to our friends and coworkers for their help and support in so many ways: Dr. Ron Seifert, Dr. Pam Dorsett, Dr. Penny Stone-Hays, Dr. Frank Batkins, Dr. Rick Blue, Sharon Wexler, Dr. Brenda Galina, Dr. Wayne Parker, Debra McElhaney, Gail Heyman, Francis Klein.

We appreciate the continuing belief that David Rosenthal and Annik La Farge, our editors at Villard Books; our literary agent Meredith Bernstein; our producers, Janet Glass and Marla Shavin of *Noonday*, WXIA-TV, demonstrate by permitting us to present our advice and views to hundreds of thousands of parents, adults, and children through the forums they represent.

CONTENTS

I

THE RITALIN
DEBATE

1

EYE OF THE STORM

Confusion and Controversy Abound

Seven-year-old **MICKEY ALVAREZ**'s *teachers suspected he might have an attention deficit hyperactivity disorder (ADHD) and referred him for testing. Like so many parents we've seen, the Alvarezes had read the headlines and had heard the terms before. Worried and confused about their son, they made their position very clear: "Don't say the R word! We won't consider giving him Ritalin."*

MR. AND MRS. COHEN *were confused. After having been diagnosed with ADHD, their eleven-year-old son* **JERALD** *had responded well to Ritalin. His teachers reported that he was able to sit at his desk for longer periods of time, completed more assignments, and generally was more attentive in class. However, his test scores had not improved significantly, nor was he getting along that much better with his parents, siblings, or classmates. Fights were still a daily occurrence. "Ritalin is no magic pill as far as we're concerned," said Mr. Cohen.*

JESSIE KELLEY *was fifteen when she came to see us. She had been diagnosed as having an attention deficit disorder when she was eight years old, had taken Ritalin, and had done quite well. Her parents were concerned because she was having difficulty paying attention and keeping up with the workload in high school. "She's a teenager now, so ADD isn't a problem anymore. What do we do?" asked her mom.*

MICHAEL PITT *is an up-and-coming lawyer. He had to struggle through law school, but made it. Although a "go-getter" and great with the tiny details of contracts, he hasn't made partner yet. When we met with him, he was beginning to wonder if he would. "I was in a* *meeting with an important client, discussing dealings that involve large sums of money. Next thing I know, I'm tracking a bird outside the window, and the client is asking me a question about I don't know what. So I bluff and tell my assistant to have the answer in the morning. I've always been this way, but I'm wondering if I could be ADD. Would Ritalin work for me?'' he asked us.*

Four different individuals; four different stories; four points of view. Depending on why you selected this book, one of these stories is likely to be yours or that of someone you know and love.

You or your child may have tried medication and found that it wasn't the magic pill you expected either. If it had some positive effects, there are probably still areas of your own behavior or your child's that concern you. Or you may have been led to believe that your child would outgrow ADHD, but it didn't happen. He's still having the same old struggles, and you wonder if Ritalin is again a possible solution.

Perhaps only recently you have come to recognize your child or yourself in the now-familiar description of ADHD individuals. Could Ritalin be the answer to your struggles? Finally, there are those of you who don't want to try any medication. You believe that your child has ADHD, but refuse to consider medication for any number of reasons.

The Alvarezes are a classic example of this last category. After they told us not to mention the *R* word, we asked why. It became clear quite quickly that, like many other parents, Mrs. Alvarez was concerned about "tranquilizing" her son. She also feared that Ritalin would stunt his growth and make him dependent on drugs. Although she didn't quite say it this way, the vehemence of her response clearly indicated she had visions of Ritalin turning her son into a short, underweight drug addict.

A much larger group of parents, upon hearing their child has an attention deficit disorder, carefully consider the pros and cons before cautiously deciding to try medication. We understand the hesitation; as parents we understand the questions associated with giving any child medication for ADHD.

Once having begun medication for ADHD, more than two thirds of the group are likely to see some improvement in the child's attention, overactivity, impulsiveness, or distractibility. However, over time parents are often surprised and disappointed, as the Cohens were, to discover that Ritalin doesn't come close to solving all their child's problems. Sometimes Ritalin initially makes such a profound difference in the life of their child that the repeated admonition, "Medication should never be the sole form of treatment for ADHD children," falls on deaf ears. Without the inclusion of a range of nonpharmaceutical interventions and techniques, medication alone in many cases is doomed, if not to fail entirely, at least to prove disappointing.

Sadly, many parents take false comfort in the old thinking that most children will "outgrow" ADHD in adolescence. Unfortunately, we know now that many individuals do not outgrow ADHD. With time, the problematic symptoms may change, or the individuals may have independently hit upon a number of coping skills, but problems and challenges remain, often requiring new adjustments and new coping techniques. More than half of ADHD children will experience adolescence as Jessica Kelley did. Old problems remain and recur in the overstimulating, hormone-surging, action-packed high school years, and the old solutions no longer work. It's never too late to try new nonpharmaceutical interventions or even medication. In fact, many ADHD teens respond well to medication, learn to accept responsibility for their actions, and ultimately find that the medication becomes crucial when they need to complete a lot of reading, or in situations demanding high attention, such as exams.

Finally, an increasing number of adults who have learned about ADHD are beginning to recognize themselves in the description. They may have struggled all their lives, may have been diagnosed with other learning disabilities, or may now be plagued by a compromised self-image based on experiences of failure and frustration. Every day we get calls from adults who, successful or struggling, wonder if medication might work for them.

OPINIONS ABOUT RITALIN

Everyone seems to have an opinion about Ritalin. Even though it is nowhere near as widely prescribed as, say, antibiotics, most of us have heard the word and know, even if only vaguely, that it is a psychoactive drug given to children who are hyperactive or have short attention spans. How Ritalin became so famous is a story unto itself. For now, though, let's suppose you are attending a lecture entitled, "Beyond Ritalin and Other Medications for ADHD." As you enter the hall, you are asked to choose one of four areas in which to sit. These are designated by signs that express the four major opinions about treating ADHD with medication:

1. No Ritalin
2. Ritalin Works, but It's No Magic Pill
3. Ritalin Used to Work, but Too Old for Medication
4. Could ADHD Be My Problem? Could Ritalin Be My Solution?

Where would you sit? Like most, you might hesitate before committing yourself to one area or another, or you might stride briskly to a particular section because you know it is right. Wherever you sit, you'll be hearing many people loudly voicing their own strong opinions about the use of medication for ADHD.

Almost every issue in life can accommodate a few reasonable points of view; answers often lie in the gray area. But for too many people, treating ADHD with medication is cast in terms of either a black-and-white yes or no, or a fog of shadowy gray that is clouded by gaps in information and blatant misconceptions. This book will give you the navigational tools you need to chart the course that's best for your child or yourself.

Those who must deal with the consequences of ADHD find the controversy surrounding it both frightening and confusing; and this complicates an already difficult decision. Sometimes the confusion and fear are so great that families and individuals simply give up and refuse to even consider any pharmaceutical intervention. We can sympathize with people who are overwhelmed by the debate and the issues, and we respect a parent's or an individual's ultimate decision. Through our years of experience with people with ADHD, however, we have seen time and again that when people base such a serious decision on insufficient, questionable, and just plain incorrect information, they immediately close the door to a range of possibilities for growth, development, and success, in school, at work, and in the rest of their lives.

We understand. After all, who wouldn't prefer clear-cut instructions when it comes to complicated issues? Who wouldn't prefer to make a decision knowing it would never be "wrong"? Pediatricians say, "Give your child the polio vaccine," and "Feed your child healthy foods." Both of these "prescriptions" clearly articulate what you should do, and we can accept them, confident that they're backed up by hard scientific data, generations of practical experience, or both.

In our experience, one of the biggest hurdles parents and individuals with ADHD face is the fact that there simply is no one "right" answer. While our knowledge about the disorder and how to treat it is expanding dramatically, ADHD remains a frustratingly multifaceted, often mysterious challenge to everyone. Medication may be one component in the treatment plan, but before you can determine that, you must seek several "right" answers through what will probably boil down to simple trial and error. Making decisions about medication is likely to make you feel as if you have been thrown into the eye of a storm. The often contradictory but passionately held opinions of professionals, family members, friends, and teachers, combined with what you read and hear, swirl loudly around you. Without a sure compass directing you to calmer waters, you venture out, anxiously bracing yourself for the next gust of wind, the next big wave.

Before you set out, understand that medication is not and can never be an end unto itself, the whole solution, the magic pill. When pressed, many people give lip service to the need for additional treatment, but in reality they essentially rely on the medication to "do it all." Whether this is simply a product of wishful thinking, professionals' failure to make this point clearly enough, or other factors is hard to say. What we do know is that in far too many instances, people do little to augment the positive effects of medication, and then are truly surprised and disappointed when the individual with ADHD continues to have problems.

This book will give you an understanding of how medication affects the individual, will outline specifically which aspects of ADHD might require additional help, and will explain what else people on medication should be doing to compensate for the characteristics of ADHD.

We are often asked to explain our position on ADHD and medication—especially Ritalin, since that is the best-known drug treatment. Simply stated, whether we or any other professionals you encounter are "for" or "against" medication for ADHD is not the issue. **What medication can and cannot do for ADHD in your case or your child's is the important question for you to ask.**

When we began working with hyperactive kids—as they were called back in the 1970s—we believed that these children could be effectively treated without medication. (Aha, you say, you knew "beyond Ritalin" meant "without Ritalin"). However, over the years many children taught us a different lesson. Medication made it possible for them to be ready for the other kinds of treatment necessary to overcome their problems. (Some of you are now sighing, "They are pro-Ritalin.") However, as we have traveled the United States, talking with parents and teachers about attention deficit hyperactivity disorder, we realized how little good, useful information they have about the specific effects of medication on ADHD.

Over and over we have heard from parents and teachers much of the same incomplete, erroneous information and misconceptions about medication and ADHD. That's not surprising if you consider how the popular media have bombarded us with hundreds of articles and television news stories about Ritalin and other medications for ADHD. What is surprising is that after so many years of use, medication for ADHD is still so grossly misunderstood.

Given what Ritalin is and what it does, it's little wonder that it attracts so much attention. Ritalin offers all the elements of a good emotional debate. The decision whether or not to put a child on ADHD medication touches upon a range of highly charged issues. For parents, the number-one concern is the health of their children. Education is number two. Fear of future drug abuse is a close third. Mix those together, then add in the money the pharmaceutical companies make from Ritalin and other medications for ADHD (leading skeptics to wonder if medication isn't overprescribed or undertested), toss in religious and ethical concerns, attach reams of sketchy information about ADHD, and you have a rousing, long-running, and, in our opinion, nonproductive controversy. Consider a few of these headlines and clippings:

RITALIN: MIRACLE OR NIGHTMARE? HYPERACTIVITY DRUG MADE ONE
BOY EXEMPLARY STUDENT, ANOTHER SCHOOL TERROR
—*Atlanta Journal and Constitution,* November 29, 1987

A sharp increase in sales of the stimulant Ritalin has rekindled an emotional debate over whether the substance is being prescribed to help youngsters with a specific hyperactivity disorder, or instead to sedate unruly pupils whom teachers cannot control.
—*The New York Times,* May 5, 1987

PARENTS AND DOCTORS FEAR GROWING MISUSE OF DRUG USED TO
TREAT HYPERACTIVE KIDS
—*The Wall Street Journal,* November 15, 1988

USE OF DRUG TO CALM CHILDREN RISES SHARPLY, STUDY REPORTS
—*Los Angeles Times,* October 21, 1988

"Researchers are raising questions about the long-term usefulness of drugs used to treat an estimated 750,000 schoolchildren nationwide for hyperactivity and inattentiveness."
—*Chicago Tribune,* October 21, 1988

. . . If misused on children without the disorder who are simply discipline problems for teachers or parents, the drugs [Ritalin] would stimu-
late, not tranquilize, them."

—The New York Times, April 25, 1991

. . . Schoolchildren are being diagnosed and medicated for the disorder [ADD] in too cavalier a fashion . . . They blame this trend on two
converging realities: the increased pressure on financially troubled
schools to provide a quick fix for disruptive children and the cutback in
mental health services. . . .

—Boston Globe, July 26, 1993

Although the effect of such media hype is strong, the controversy
about the use of stimulant medication was truly propelled into the lime-
light during the 1980s, when several lawsuits were filed by parents contending that Ritalin had harmed their children. One Georgia mother
alleged that Ritalin caused her sixteen-year-old son to suffer physical
retardation and brain damage. Although the suit was dropped, the controversy did not end. Reports of a teenager committing suicide after taking Ritalin for nine years, and three other students committing suicide
after being treated for hyperactivity with the antidepressant medication
Norpramin, further frightened and confused the public.

Ritalin *was* big news. Some charged that special-interest groups,
which may have had their own larger agendas having little to do with
the treatment of ADHD, promoted misconceptions and fallacies about
Ritalin. For example, according to the *Los Angeles Times*, several groups
such as the Citizens Commission on Human Rights, located in Los Angeles, used the media to wage a war against Ritalin. The *Los Angeles Times*
reported on June 29, 1990, that "While alerting parents and teachers to
the dangers of Ritalin, the real target of the campaign is the psychiatric
profession itself."

Heightened concerns about misdiagnosis and overuse were reinforced by frequent articles cataloging the growing use of Ritalin. Articles
in *The New York Times, The Boston Globe, The Atlanta Journal and Constitution*, the *Los Angeles Times, USA Today*, and other newspapers tracked increased percentages of prescriptions for Ritalin, especially in the South.
Other articles alarmed parents with reports of possible shortages of the
drug.

Here was a burning controversy that generated a tremendous
amount of heat and plenty of sparks, but precious little light. The popular

media coverage of Ritalin and ADHD has contributed only a drop of hard, reliable information, while fanning the flames of concern, fear, anger, and confusion among professionals, parents, and those who have ADHD. Most recently, a report by the Food and Drug Administration of a possible link between cancer and ingestion of thirty times the normal dose of Ritalin by rats roused concern. Although the FDA stated there was no evidence of risk to humans and no reason to take Ritalin off the market, fear remains. The fact that Ritalin use by children and adolescents has been studied for more than thirty years with no link to harmful disease has not been reported as strongly.

It's often said that no one forgets a first impression, and this seems particularly true for Ritalin and other medications for ADHD. The many excellent books written by professionals who diligently set forth facts about the role of medication in the treatment of ADHD and the efforts to bring to light new scientific data are no match for the sensationalized, oversimplified avalanche of misinformation. The public's initial response of mistrust and confusion often remains unchanged. In the meantime, untold children and adults who could benefit from the proper use of medication in conjunction with a range of behavioral and organizational techniques are forgoing medication and suffering needlessly.

Considering how complicated attention deficit hyperactivity disorder is and how frustrating it is for those trying to live with it, it is crucial that individuals have *all* the facts. And that brings us to our position on medication for ADHD:

ADHD is a complex disorder. It cannot simply be cured by a pill. It is crucial for ADHD youngsters and adults, their loved ones, and those who work with them to understand what effect medication may have on the troubling characteristics of the disorder. If they elect to use medication, they must realize that it is never the sole form of treatment, and they must make the commitment to identify and work to control, cope with, or solve those problems that medication alone simply cannot solve.

FINDING THE FACTS ABOUT ADHD

Start with the name. What is ADHD? Does it refer to the same problems as ADD, or ADD/H?

Beginning with Fidgety Phil, as it was known in the early part of the century, and moving through hyperactivity, attention deficit disorder (ADD), ADD with and without hyperactivity (ADD/H), and the more recent ADHD, the various labels assigned to this disorder reflect changes in the emphasis placed on its various characteristics. More recent names—such as ADHD, ADHD inattentive type, impulsive type combined, or others—reflect an increasing awareness that the disorder has various subtypes that play out in different ways and combinations for each individual. Further, how ADHD manifests in a single individual may change over time.

Although the terms ADD and ADHD popularly refer to the same disorder, for the purposes of this book we most often use the shorthand initials ADHD when discussing "the disorder." Elsewhere in the book we will identify each specific characteristic of ADHD, how medication may affect it, and what else can be done to influence the characteristic.

Obviously, our understanding of the disorder has undergone numerous major overhauls. Science has speculated about the causes of ADHD for decades, but only recently, with the help of high-tech imaging devices such as PET scans and magnetic resonance imaging (MRI), has the disorder been shown to have a verifiable physical cause. Despite thousands of research studies about ADHD, however, it takes a dedicated effort to extract conclusions about the effects of medication on the disorder. Furthermore, the specific outcomes remain largely unpredictable and unique to each individual. This is why it takes a team approach on the part of several people to ascertain how well medication is working in each case.

In the following chapter, *Beyond Ritalin* will correct the misconceptions associated with the use of Ritalin and other medications to treat ADHD. The rest of the book presents a clear discussion of what medication does and does not do to attention, self-control, learning, social skills, organization, and other aspects of attention deficit hyperactivity disorder.

Having the facts about the effects of medication on ADHD and the individual should allow you to make an informed decision about whether and when it is feasible to try medication. Also, understanding what aspects of ADHD medication might improve gives you a frame of reference for determining what other treatments are important to your situation. With facts in hand, *Beyond Ritalin* will empower you to steer out of the eye of the storm to help your child or yourself succeed in overcoming the problems associated with ADHD.

2

MEDICATION MYTHS

Facts and Fallacies About Medication

It could be the basis of a television game show or a category of questions in Trivial Pursuit: "Facts and Fallacies about Ritalin." However, the truth or consequences of this misinformation are no game. Misunderstandings about medication prevent some parents from giving a child who is having extreme difficulty in the classroom the help that medication can offer to some ADHD individuals. When properly administered and monitored, medication enables some children and adults to sit still longer and to be more attentive so each is more ready to learn, read, act and do.

On the other hand, relying completely and solely on Ritalin to solve the complicated problems of ADHD reflects an incomplete understanding of what role medication can play in the treatment of ADHD. Believing, erroneously, that medication is a "miracle pill" that cures ADHD can result in disappointment, frustration, and worse.

Even the best-informed individuals may have picked up some faulty information about ADHD and medication. Where do you fit in? Take this little quiz to determine your level of knowledge about medication and ADHD. Circle *T* or *F* after reading each statement, and then read on to find out which statements are myths and which are not.

True or False about ADHD

1. By causing either a decline in appetite or a permanent suppression of growth hormone, medication for ADHD stunts a child's growth.   T   F

2. Stimulants like Ritalin are the only medications used in the treatment of ADHD.   T   F

3. There is a standard dosage for each medication that is based on a person's weight.   T   F

4. Ritalin causes children and adults to be more aggressive.   T   F

5. Children and adults who take Ritalin or other medication for ADHD are more likely to abuse psychoactive drugs and alcohol.   T   F

6. Anyone with a history of drug dependency should not take medication for ADHD.   T   F

7. Ritalin and other medications lose their effectiveness when a child reaches puberty.   T   F

8. Medication works equally well on all aspects of ADHD.   T   F

9. Too many children are being placed on medication for ADHD.   T   F

10. Ritalin and other medications for ADHD are "miracle drugs."   T   F

11. ADHD affects only someone's ability to learn; there's no harm in ceasing medication when there's no school or work to attend to.   T   F

12. Trying a course of Ritalin or other medication for ADHD is the best way to confirm a diagnosis.   T   F

13. The effects of Ritalin and other medication for ADHD are clearly understood and always predictable.   T   F

14. Medication is the only effective treatment for ADHD.   T   F

DISPELLING THE MYTHS ABOUT MEDICATION

MYTH #1: MEDICATION FOR ADHD STUNTS A CHILD'S GROWTH.

No drug, not even those we generally consider safe, such as aspirin, is without side effects. That is why pharmacists in many states are now required to offer counseling about possible side effects and proper use of every drug they prescribe.

While there are many side effects associated with Ritalin, most of them, including irritability, ease of crying, and anxiety, are also associated with ADHD itself. In fact, studies, including one by Dr. Russell Barkley, probably the best-known and most highly esteemed researcher on ADHD, indicate that mood-related side effects such as these are also reported by parents on days when Ritalin is replaced with a placebo.

Ritalin, in particular, is generally considered to be a well-researched, safe medication with few long-term side effects. Ritalin does not permanently suppress a child's growth, although some children may experience reduced appetite. Practically speaking, many parents are able to get around the appetite effects of medication by adjusting the time of dosage until after meals. Further concerns about growth can be allayed by "drug holidays," a recess when the child temporarily takes a break from medication. The research literature indicates growth rebounds often occur during such "holidays."

Appetite suppression and insomnia, two well-documented side effects of Ritalin or its generic equivalent, methylphenidate, appear to be dose-related. This is especially true for dextroamphetamine or Dexedrine. The higher the dosage, the greater the effect for more than one half of the children studied. Follow-up research indicates that most appetite reduction and any accompanying growth suppression occur during the first year of treatment. Happily, though, these effects do not appear to be long-lasting. Children tend to rebound during the second year of medication use, and Ritalin usage itself seems to have no significant effect on ultimate adult height and weight.

Weight and size were especially important to ten-year-old Jim S. when we first diagnosed his ADHD in 1983. He was an athlete and wanted to build bulk and muscle so he could play high school football. Over the years he continued to take Ritalin to help with his severe ADHD problems, and practiced weight lifting. As Jim grew and grew we ultimately decided it was more appropriate to call him "Mr. S." Medication helped him concentrate in school, and you certainly couldn't tell him from the rest of the team size-wise. Reduced appetite and growth suppression did not occur with this youngster.

Of course, if you have a child who is ADHD and small for his age, you naturally will worry about this issue. However, our experience both personally and professionally has been that many children like this are finicky eaters. Once a finicky eater, always a finicky eater—at least during childhood. Medication is not likely to change that one way or the other.

On the other side of the weight and height issue, a number of parents who have said, "Perhaps Ritalin will help with my child's overweight problem," did not find this to be the case either. Ironically, heavier children did not lose any noticeable pounds while on Ritalin.

It is extremely important for any child taking any medication to be monitored by a physician, which means having your doctor periodically review your child's weight and growth during the course of medication and compare it with his long-term growth pattern. If any modifications of medical treatment need to be made, your physician will be able to do so.

MYTH #2: STIMULANTS ARE THE ONLY MEDICATIONS USED IN THE TREATMENT OF ADHD.

The answer to question two of our quiz is definitely False. Although stimulants are the best-known medications used to treat ADHD, many children have been treated successfully with other medications.

As you know by now, Ritalin is the best-known and most widely used treatment for ADHD. More children take Ritalin or its generic equivalent, methylphenidate, for the treatment of ADHD than any other drug for any other childhood disorder. In fact, up to 750,000 U.S. children are reported to take Ritalin daily.

There are, however, several other central nervous system stimulants that are also widely prescribed for this disorder. These include Ritalin SR, a time-release form of methylphenidate, Dexedrine or dextroamphetamine (d-amphetamine), and Cylert or pemoline. (See Chapter 5, "When Medication Is Needed," for further discussion of each named medication or its generic equivalent.)

Numerous research studies have documented the positive short-term effects of stimulant medication on behavior, social interactions, and academic functioning for the children who take them. We can blame the media for erroneously using "Ritalin" as a universal term for ADHD medications.

Aside from the stimulants, a number of other kinds of medication have shown beneficial effects on ADHD. Tricyclic antidepressants such as desipramine and imipramine are slower-acting medications that have been reported by teachers to improve attention, activity level, and aggression among more than two thirds of the ADHD students treated with antidepressants. However, there is no evidence that antidepressants improve cognitive performance on the vigilance tasks typically used to assess sustained attention in ADHD children. On the downside, their side effects include increases in blood pressure and heart rate as well as possible slowing of intracardiac conduction. Antidepressants require more intense monitoring than is typically necessary for stimulants. Thus, for most ADHD children, stimulants are favored because of their superior positive effects. However, for those individuals who do not respond to stimulant medication, antidepressants may be a promising alternative.

Future research may provide additional pharmaceutical alternatives for ADHD children. The literature reports studies of small samples of children where monoamine oxidase inhibitors and the anticonvulsant clonidine have been found to be very effective in treating hyperactivity and conduct problems.

MYTH #3: A PERSON'S WEIGHT DETERMINES THE STANDARD DOSAGE FOR EACH MEDICATION.

Not true. There is no magic dosage that works for all children or adults.

Ritalin is most often prescribed in 2.5 mg increments, with an individual dose beginning at 5.0 mg. Weight does not appear to be the optimum determinant of the best-fit dosage. Two children of the same age and weight may respond quite differently to the same dose of Ritalin. One may experience no apparent effect while the other may report increased attention and ability to control movement. A larger child may respond positively to a lower dosage, and a child of lesser weight may require a larger dosage to gain the same positive effects.

The typical practice with Ritalin is to initially prescribe a low dose of 5 mg once a day. On the basis of feedback from "the team"—in the child's case that would include the child, parents, individual teachers, physician, and therapist—the medication would be adjusted until a therapeutic effect is noted.

Marc presents a typical case. Marc's pediatrician began with a trial dose of 5 mg in the morning. After reports from family and teachers, he recommended that Marc also take 5 mg of Ritalin at noon. Further feedback led the physician to increase the medication by 2.5 mg increments until a positive response was noted. The proper dosage for this child of eight turned out to be 10 mg in the morning before leaving for school and 7.5 mg at noon. A full discussion of the proper use of medication is presented in Chapter 5.

MYTH #4: RITALIN CAUSES CHILDREN AND ADULTS TO BE AGGRESSIVE.

No! Ritalin does not *cause* aggression. In fact, low and moderate dosages of Ritalin have been found to reduce aggression. There are reports, though, that Ritalin causes some individuals to feel edgy or irritable. Since these are characteristics of ADHD anyway, it is tricky to attribute irritability and fluctuating emotions to the medication. In addition, if a child or adult, especially one who is already experiencing frustration, is feeling irritable, then she might be more likely to respond to certain situations in a more aggressive manner.

A side effect associated with Ritalin that may contribute to this myth is the "behavioral rebound" effect associated with methylphenidate and other medications. About a third of the children taking Ritalin become more irritable, and their behavior becomes more difficult to control, as medication wears off. Typically, this occurs in the late afternoon as the noon dose of medication taken at school is wearing off. It's interesting to note that the rebound effect doesn't occur consistently in most children, and most of the time the effect is lessened by administering a reduced dose of medication in the late afternoon, or by decreasing the noon dosage.

MYTH #5: CHILDREN AND ADULTS WHO TAKE ADHD MEDICATION ARE MORE LIKELY TO ABUSE DRUGS AND ALCOHOL.

This does appear to be a myth, although it is harder to provide a definitive response to this statement. The conventional wisdom is the following: ADHD individuals are naturally impulsive. They are prone to rush headfirst into a number of situations without regard to the consequences. When an ADHD youth gets involved with drugs, it is the disorder and *not* the medication the child is taking that puts him at risk. ADHD youth who take stimulant medications that have a positive effect on behavior are often better able to cope with the pressures of growing up and are less likely to turn to drugs.

All of the above is true, yet the research in this area is somewhat confusing. Some studies have found that ADHD adolescents are more likely to try drugs, most notably nonprescription and illegal drugs, than their peers. This is especially true of those who did not receive consistent treatment for ADHD and who have also been diagnosed with a conduct disorder. A study conducted by Russell Barkley and reported in his book *Attention Deficit Hyperactivity Disorder,* which carefully controlled for teens who were solely ADHD and who did not have other conduct disorders, found that ADHD youth are no more likely to use cigarettes or alcohol than their "normal" counterparts. The general consensus is that although ADHD youth might try marijuana, hallucinogens, and other street drugs on impulse, they are no more likely to become abusers than the rest of the population.

Adolescents and adults who have undiagnosed ADHD are often frustrated, depressed, and unhappy. They may feel anxious or angry. They're likely to feel "scattered" or unfocused and turn to drugs to "self-medicate." Interestingly, a number of adult abusers of cocaine who are also ADHD report that the drug made them feel focused rather than high. Alcohol and marijuana can do much the same thing, lessening the discomfort and "noise" many adults associate with ADHD.

The recent reports by the media about the abuse of Ritalin by high school and college students have increased parental concern that taking Ritalin for ADHD may lead to later illicit drug use. The media reports about the abuse of Ritalin fail to emphasize that it was the use of Ritalin by non-ADHD students to get high that is claimed to be on the rise. If it is true that drugs fill an immediate need or look appealing to the untreated ADHD youth or adult, then dealing with ADHD early on would seem even more imperative in light of this information. Unfortunately, there is no guarantee that treating your child for ADHD will "inoculate" her against future drug use. Given the decades-long "drug crisis," it's safe to say that nothing can do that. However, it is unlikely that the act of taking Ritalin or another medication for ADHD will contribute to or increase a child's risk for later drug use.

MYTH #6: ANYONE WITH A HISTORY OF DRUG DEPENDENCY
SHOULD NOT TAKE MEDICATION FOR ADHD.

The question of whether to prescribe Ritalin for a previously undiagnosed ADHD adult who has a history of drug abuse is also a complicated
decision. It is important not to automatically assume that the individual
should *never* be treated with medication. Treating ADHD with medication
alone is a mistake for anyone, regardless of previous drug history. However, stimulants such as Ritalin, when carefully monitored and used in
coordination with treatment for the characteristics of ADHD *and* drug
abuse, may provide the organized, balanced effort and support the individual needs to avoid other drugs and to feel better about himself.

MYTH #7: RITALIN AND OTHER MEDICATIONS LOSE THEIR
EFFECTIVENESS WHEN A CHILD REACHES PUBERTY.

False. The popular position used to be that children would outgrow
ADHD during puberty; hence, the conclusion that medications lose
their effectiveness at that time. We now know that more than one
half of ADHD children do not outgrow the disorder. Hyperactive behavior is likely to lessen, but for most youngsters, ADHD symptoms continue.

Studies conducted over the last twenty years consistently indicate
that most individuals do not outgrow ADHD. If you are one of the increasing number of previously undiagnosed adults with ADHD who are
seeking help from professionals, you know this.

While it is untrue that Ritalin and other stimulant medications become ineffective after an ADHD youth passes through puberty, the
amount of medication needed to manage ADHD symptoms may change
for a number of reasons. The demands on the individual change, the
youth's ability to cope with the characteristics of ADHD hopefully improves, and, of course, changes in body size, weight, and metabolism
alter how the body processes medication.

As teenagers learn to manage the symptoms of ADHD, they may be
able to function effectively on lower dosages of medication. One youth
whom we worked with off and on for years went off medication during
early adolescence. Not wanting to be different from his peers, he preferred to stop all medication. This worked well for a while. As the demands of academics and extracurricular activities began to overwhelm

him in college, he decided medication would help him to focus better and to use his time more wisely.

MYTH #8: MEDICATION WORKS EQUALLY WELL ON ALL ASPECTS OF ADHD.

No, absolutely not. Medication does not solve all aspects of ADHD. You have watched your child struggle, or have struggled yourself, with the remaining effects of ADHD. Perhaps medication does allow you or your child to attend longer, to focus better, and to inhibit some responses. Your child's handwriting may improve and he may complete his assignments in a more timely fashion—if he remembers to take them to school. Your daughter may be less fidgety, or you may be better able to sit through staff meetings. However, you may be continually surprised to see that your child's overall level of achievement has not improved. While your child may be more compliant and less aggressive with peers, may even get along better with siblings, he may not seem to be more social or better liked. No, medication doesn't cure or even take care of all the difficult characteristics an ADHD child or adult may experience.

MYTH #9: TOO MANY CHILDREN ARE BEING PLACED ON MEDICATION FOR ADHD.

False. The newspaper headlines would have you believe otherwise, but the hard, scientific statistics read differently.

The overall number of children who have ADHD is conservatively placed at 3 to 5 percent of the childhood population, or one in every twenty-five to thirty children. This adds up to over 2 million children in the United States who have been diagnosed with ADHD.

Depending on the study, the estimates of the number of children being treated with Ritalin range from 750,000 to 1.6 million youngsters. These numbers are substantially less than the estimated population of children with the disorder.

The percentage of children treated with Ritalin in a particular location, however, does vary. A study of use of Ritalin in Michigan found that the number of boys taking Ritalin for ADHD ranged from 1 percent to 10 percent, depending on the county in which they lived. The number of Massachusetts schoolchildren on Ritalin in 1993 was 4,836, or 0.6 percent of the school-age children. In Georgia, which has been attacked for having one of the highest rates of Ritalin use in the South, 3.5 percent of the total population of children are estimated to take Ritalin. Although these figures may correspond to socioeconomic class or other factors that influence incidence, none of these numbers is out of line with the population generally believed to be ADHD.

The important question, then, should be not how many children are on medication for ADHD or even whether too many children are taking Ritalin, but whether medication is appropriate for the individual child, and what other treatments must be coordinated with medication.

MYTH #10: RITALIN AND OTHER MEDICATIONS FOR ADHD ARE "MIRACLE CURES."

False, although for a few individuals, the effects of Ritalin or another medication may be so dramatic that a miracle seems to have occurred. For most children and adults, however, the effects of medication are more subtle. As we've said before, medication is not a cure for ADHD or the myriad problems often associated with it.

MYTH #11: THERE'S NO NEED FOR ADHD MEDICATION OR OTHER INTERVENTIONS OUTSIDE SCHOOL AND WORK SITUATIONS.

False. As we know, ADHD can have a significant adverse effect on the skills and abilities that facilitate learning. But we also know the same characteristics of inattention and impulsiveness that make learning or working difficult for someone with ADHD can have a negative impact in social situations. As a result, ADHD children and adults often have trouble making and keeping friends, adjusting to changes, and following routines. This is true whether they are in the classroom, on the football field, or at home. Thus, some individuals will benefit from taking medication at times other than formal learning or work situations.

MYTH #12: TRYING RITALIN OR OTHER MEDICATION IS THE BEST WAY TO CONFIRM A DIAGNOSIS.

False. Although we dedicate an entire chapter to this topic (Chapter 3), we feel it's important to note here that this dangerous misconception is still held by some. There are many steps to obtaining an accurate diagnosis of ADHD, which we outline in the next chapter; trying a course of medication in search of the "paradoxical effect" is most definitely not one of them. Be highly suspicious of any professional who suggests otherwise.

MYTH #13: THE EFFECTS OF RITALIN AND OTHER MEDICATIONS FOR ADHD ARE CLEARLY UNDERSTOOD AND ALWAYS PREDICTABLE.

Even medications that have been thoroughly tested for safety sometimes work in ways that remain something of a mystery—even to the companies that produce them and the doctors who prescribe them. This is particularly true of psychoactive drugs, a group that includes Ritalin and other ADHD medications. Further, because ADHD is a multifaceted, complex disorder, each individual's response to medication will be unique and impossible to predict. The process of trial and error required before the right drug in the right dosage taken on the right schedule is determined is perhaps one of the more frustrating aspects for people with ADHD and those trying to help them. If it's any consolation, you must remember that it is rarely simple, and the positive benefits of working hard to find the right fit may reward your efforts.

MYTH #14: MEDICATION IS THE ONLY EFFECTIVE TREATMENT FOR ADHD.

Absolutely false. Some people with ADHD live full, productive lives without ever taking medication; others find that they need it to help them overcome a range of difficulties. We've said this before, but the point cannot be overemphasized: There is no one simple solution to ADHD. Virtually anyone with ADHD needs to adopt at least a few and perhaps many of the behavioral, organizational, and social practices we present throughout this book. In some cases, altering environments, shifting schedules, and integrating a host of behavior modifiers into one's daily schedule will be enough to render medication unnecessary. It's important to remember that medication can neither replace nor do the work of nonpharmaceutical alternatives. Medication cannot teach a student how to read, nor can it remind a salesman to make phone calls. What it often can do is to set the stage, so to speak, making it possible for people with ADHD to better cope with the challenges they face.

A FINAL WORD ON MYTHS ABOUT MEDICATION

We hope this chapter has cleared up some of the common misconceptions about medication. No matter how often they are repeated or by whom, all of these statements are false.

Clearing your path of misconceptions, myths, and erroneous information should be your first step. Understanding the facts about medication and ADHD gives you a head start on making the decisions that will be important to you or your child.

II

BEYOND RITALIN

3

WHY RITALIN DOESN'T DIAGNOSE ADHD

How to Get an Accurate Diagnosis

The fact that your performance improves when you take Ritalin doesn't mean that you are ADHD.
The fact that you do not respond to Ritalin doesn't mean that you are not ADHD.

One of the most serious misconceptions surrounding Ritalin is the assumption that this medication can be used as a litmus test to determine if a person has ADHD. Many people, both professionals and laypersons, have assumed that a positive response to Ritalin or another medication is "proof" that the individual has the disorder. Similarly, the opposite is also presumed to be accurate; that is, no response to a medication indicates the person does not have ADHD. Over the past decade, a great amount of research evidence contradicts both points of view.

THE MYTH OF THE PARADOXICAL EFFECT

The notion of using responses to medication to diagnose ADHD sprang from the belief that people with ADD/hyperactivity disorder would somehow react differently from so-called normal individuals. It was a view that was not based on scientifically controlled studies; rather, it evolved from the observation that hyperactive children seem to calm down when given a stimulant.

Of course, the notion of "stimulating" an already overactive child flies in the face of common sense. Thus, the only reasonable explanation would appear to be some sort of "paradoxical," or reverse, effect. Justification for the paradoxical effect began to crumble in 1980, when Dr. Judy Rapoport and her colleagues at the National Institute of Mental Health conducted a landmark experiment. Both ADD/hyperactive and "normal" children were given stimulants under well-controlled conditions. The researchers then measured both cognitive and behavioral effects of the medication. Surprisingly, *both* groups performed better on medication. Therefore, there was no paradoxical effect: Everyone— ADHD or not—performed better on stimulant medication!

The Rapoport study has been replicated several times. If you think about it, the fact that most people performed better on stimulants is not so surprising. How often have you reached for a cup of coffee when you felt a little drowsy? You also probably know a couple of college students who took a few "uppers" to concentrate better so they could cram for exams. You've read about how truck drivers, train engineers, and others who work long, tedious hours take amphetamines to "stay on the job." As a society, we constantly use psychoactive stimulants such as caffeine and nicotine to give us a "pick-me-up."

Stimulants clearly help many individuals think more clearly, concentrate better, and maintain alertness. That is, until they become overmedicated. Then a person may seem drugged or sluggish. Some non-ADHD children and adults may reach this state more quickly, but response to medication is unique to each individual and very difficult to predict.

None of this totally repudiates the "paradoxical effect." Since most people think of stimulants as drugs that rev up the body, the fact that both individuals with ADD characteristics and those who don't have them perform better on stimulants remains somewhat confusing. This is especially true if you maintain that ADHD is about hyperactivity.

How can a stimulant calm an overactive child? Isn't that a paradoxical effect? It certainly looks like one.

In the early part of this century ADHD was considered a problem of activity level. These children were unable to control their behavior. That's true for many ADHD children. However, on the basis of the work of Dr. Virginia Douglas and her colleagues at McGill University, it has long been recognized that people with this problem have difficulty with attention. Anything that helps these children and adults attend better and concentrate more easily will also allow them to have better control of their activity level.

Consider this situation: You are sitting in a large auditorium. It is very warm and the seats are completely filled. The speaker is reading his paper on a devastatingly boring topic. You cannot leave, but you must look interested. What do you do? Unless you are superhuman, you probably begin squirming. You may find yourself restlessly turning in your seat, moving your feet, playing with your fingers, daydreaming, and straining to keep your eyes open.

Consider a second situation. Same room. You are listening to a fascinating speaker with great theatrical flair tell a series of entertaining anecdotes. Your eyes are riveted on his face. It's still warm in the room, but you hardly notice. Your body is comfortably still as you soak up the tales being told.

What changed? You have no trouble maintaining your attention in the latter situation. And for as long as your mind is fully engaged, your activity level is very low. This is similar to what you can observe when an ADHD youth is watching TV or playing a video game. Sometimes such youngsters are so overfocused when engaged in these types of activities that they hardly move and aren't even aware of what is happening around them.

In a very simplified manner, stimulants help ADHD individuals engage their minds and attention. Activity levels drop because they are able to concentrate and inhibit motor responses. Is this a paradoxical effect? Apparently not. The same seems to be true for everyone.

MEDICATION IS NOT A DIAGNOSTIC TOOL

After reviewing the literature on medication of children with ADHD, Drs. Carol Whalen and Barbara Henker of the University of California, in a 1991 study, concluded that if any group of parents and their offspring, both ADHD and not, were to participate in a controlled trial of stimulant medication, many of the parents and the children would show significant improvements in their ability to concentrate and to complete tasks, regardless of whether a diagnosis of ADHD was appropriate. In other words, stimulants can work for anyone, and are not a valid diagnostic device.

The results of both the Rapoport and the Whalen/Henker studies undermine the rationale many professionals have employed to place children and adults on medication before a standard diagnosis has been completed. Unfortunately, a child's positive response to ADHD medication is still too often read as definitive proof that the decision to use medication was correct. Some professionals also "deduce" from a positive response that the *dosage* is correct as well. The facts, however, are to the contrary. Correct dosages of medication are often not found immediately, and follow-up monitoring is often infrequent.

In 1987 Dr. Linda Copeland of Foundation Health, Sacramento, California, found that almost 40 percent of the pediatricians she surveyed used no standardized diagnostic measures before placing children on medication for ADHD-like symptoms. The rest used rating scales from parents and teachers to make the same decision. For 73 percent of the doctors, the parents' report of the child's response to medication was rated as a very important source of information for determining if medication was working. Yet parents typically do not see the direct effects of medication while the child is at school. Follow-up ratings from teachers were less often obtained by the physicians.

Besides the obviously misguided fact-finding on the part of these physicians, there is another troubling aspect to the results of this study. Normal children have been shown to respond positively to stimulants, and as many as 20 to 30 percent of children with ADHD may not. Therefore, non-ADHD children who responded positively to the medication could be misdiagnosed as ADHD, and a negative response from an ADHD child could result in no treatment. On a more positive note, Dr. Copeland found that pediatricians trained since 1970 were much more likely to employ more complete diagnostic procedures in assessing ADHD.

AVOIDING THE WRONG DIAGNOSIS

The wrong diagnosis can lead to many kinds of problems. The two major diagnostic errors you want to avoid are:

1. False Positive

This occurs when an individual's behavior improves on medication and he is therefore diagnosed ADHD, *but* the diagnosis is wrong.

ROBERT *is an animated fourth-grader who is having trouble following directions and completing his work in school. In second grade, he was started on Ritalin and it seemed to help "for a while." His medication was increased several times in third and fourth grades. His doctor even tried several other medications. Since Robert continued to struggle in school, his doctor and teacher referred him for a complete psychoeducational assessment.*

Testing showed that Robert has significant variations in abilities and processing problems that are associated with learning disabilities. Considering his significant processing problems, one might conclude that Robert's attention and concentration are quite good. However, since he is several years behind in reading and written expression, he needs special education, not medication.

Robert's story demonstrates the merits of a detailed psychoeducational evaluation. While medication appeared to lead to an improvement in performance, and therefore was judged as effective, in reality, it masked a very different underlying problem.

The unfortunate outcome of misdiagnosis is that the individual often struggles for a long time before the truth surfaces. In the meantime, the student does not master necessary skills, experiences repeated failures, and develops a poor self-image.

There are a number of other reasons why a child at school or an adult at work might have difficulty sustaining concentration or completing tasks. Getting an accurate diagnosis means ruling out medical, psychological, and learning problems that can interfere with concentration and can block learning and work completion.

2. False Negative

This occurs when an individual is not diagnosed ADHD because he does not respond to stimulants, yet the individual is, in fact, ADHD.

CHERYL *is twenty, but still a freshman in college and flunking out. When she came in for testing to find out why, she stated, "It can't be ADD. I was given Ritalin in fourth grade and it didn't help." She spent most of high school daydreaming, yet was bright enough to "get by." However, in college she can't make it through a lecture or concentrate long enough in the library to read even part of an assignment. During the assessment, in the quiet of our office, she was easily distracted by pictures on the wall, sounds from the hallway, and her thoughts. It took Cheryl two days to complete tests that most people finish in one day. Test* *results confirmed that she has an attention deficit hyperactivity disorder, inattentive type.*

Cheryl's story demonstrates the importance of not using Ritalin as a diagnostic tool. She had and continues to have all the classic symptoms of ADHD, but she did not show any improvement when given Ritalin. Other individuals may show response or partial response to medications, but without significant improvement. Concluding that these individuals are not ADHD can have devastating, lifelong consequences. The correct conclusion is that Ritalin does not work for these individuals, not that they definitely do not have ADHD.

Ritalin is not a diagnostic tool. Neither is Dexedrine, Cylert, or any medication that may be given to treat ADHD. It is important to keep in mind that response to medication is an individual matter and is unpredictable. Although 75 to 80 percent of people properly diagnosed with attention deficit disorder respond to the first stimulant tried, as many as 20 percent don't show any improvement or have an adverse reaction. Many will respond to a second medication, but a number of individuals who are diagnosed with ADHD will not respond to any drug. This does not mean that the diagnosis is in error.

HOW TO GET AN ACCURATE DIAGNOSIS

Unfortunately, there is no single test that can identify whether you or your child has ADHD. In fact, getting an accurate diagnosis requires skillful detective work by you, your doctor or psychologist, and possibly other professionals. Although this may sound complicated, it won't be if you take it one step at a time.

Through the rest of this chapter, we will outline the steps to a complete, correct diagnosis. As you make your way through, always remember that you are your child's and your own best advocate. Ultimately, whatever decision you reach should be your own. That's why it is important for you to understand this process and the types of information you want to gather. A label of ADHD is only a rough sketch. As you accumulate valuable information during this process, you'll see how each new bit of knowledge fills in the picture, giving you a fuller understanding of the problems that are unique to your situation so the best treatment program can be designed to address them.

STEP 1. READ ABOUT THE DIFFERENT TYPES OF MEDICAL, PSYCHOLOGICAL, AND LEARNING PROBLEMS THAT MAY MIMIC ADHD.

The Diagnostic Checklist on page 52 will help ensure you have covered all of the bases. Use the symptom list as you talk with your doctor to determine what types of tests need to be done.

STEP 2. RULE OUT MEDICAL PROBLEMS.

Make an appointment for a complete examination by your physician to eliminate medical problems that could mimic ADHD or affect concentration. If you or your child has had a thorough physical exam within the last year, that is usually sufficient. After reviewing the questions in the Diagnostic Checklist, you may have a few specific questions you will want to bring to your doctor's attention. However, if you or your child is showing recent changes in behavior or symptoms, an updated exam is recommended.

Explain to your doctor why you are there and what your concerns are. During the physical, the doctor will screen for a number of conditions. Depending on what your physician finds, she may refer you to a specialist. Some of the conditions that will be considered include vision and hearing problems, thyroid problems, allergies, neurological problems, and others. A brief discussion of each follows.

Vision Problems

It doesn't happen very often, but over the years we have discovered a number of children, teenagers, and adults whose problems with attention are due to vision problems. Today fewer than one third of the states in the United States require vision screening by schools. Typically, a child doesn't have a clue that his vision differs from his peers'. Why should he if that's the way he has always seen?

This oversight can happen to anyone. An eight-year-old girl was sent to us for evaluation because she was not completing her schoolwork and was spending an inordinate amount of class time daydreaming. During testing, we noticed that she positioned her paper and held her head in an unusual way as she wrote. After an eye examination by a specialist, she was found to be farsighted and almost legally blind in one eye. Her parents were horrified to learn that she had such significant undiagnosed vision problems.

Another child we worked with, a ten-year-old boy who had trouble copying from the board and who was reportedly "hyperactive" during morning "board work," turned out to be nearsighted. He knew he couldn't see the board but had chosen not to share the information because he didn't want to wear eyeglasses.

It's alarming to note, but according to Prevent Blindness America (formerly the National Society to Prevent Blindness), one in twenty preschool children and one in four school-age students have eye problems. But don't assume that children are the only ones with undiscovered eye problems. A young college student who presumed he had outgrown his astigmatism met with us, complaining he had a short attention span. He offhandedly mentioned he sometimes saw "floating words" and experienced eye fatigue after reading for even short periods of time. The original eye problems were reconfirmed by his ophthalmologist.

Parents are often the first ones to identify vision problems. The list of symptoms of visual difficulties presented in Table 3.1 will provide a help-

---

Table 3.1
Symptoms of Vision Difficulties

_____ Dizziness, headaches, nausea after reading or writing.

_____ Clumsiness and lack of coordination with small motor tasks such as tying shoes and zipping or buttoning clothing.

_____ Rubbing eyes, blinking excessively, exhibiting sensitivity to light.

_____ Unusual turn of head or repeated effort to hold paper in just the right position.

_____ Preferring to sit very close to or far away from source of material.

_____ Difficulties at school in completing work, seeing blackboard.

_____ Complaints about looking at computer screen or following along in text.

ful clue if your child does have a vision problem. Of course, you will have to go to an eye specialist for an examination. Have him or her check for nearsightedness, farsightedness, astigmatism, and color blindness. Also check for focusing or tracking problems.

Hearing Difficulties

Many children and adolescents we evaluate have a history of frequent ear infections. Sometimes the infections are so severe that hearing is temporarily affected, leaving gaps in the child's language development or learning.

As they get older, some children continue to have fluctuations in hearing due to congestion from colds and allergies that may also interfere with learning in school settings. Still others have good auditory acuity but have difficulty discriminating certain sounds, so that they cannot distinguish between similar-sounding pairs of words or letters, or may be unable to separate background noise from the foreground. All of these hearing-related difficulties can interfere with a student's ability to understand and follow oral directions and instruction, and this can make the student appear inattentive.

Your doctor can do a hearing screening to determine if additional audiological and speech/language assessments are needed. A psychologist or language specialist can screen for language-processing problems. Some symptoms of hearing difficulties are presented in Table 3.2.

Table 3.2
Symptoms of Hearing Difficulties

_____ Continually turning head toward sound or speaker.
_____ Frequently mishearing conversation.
_____ Difficulty with oral directions.
_____ Frequently interrupting other speakers.
_____ Difficulty differentiating between similar words or sounds.
_____ Other speech and language problems.

Thyroid Problems

Although it is rare for thyroid problems to cause attentional difficulties, it can happen. We will always remember the call from a young man in Minneapolis to a radio talk show on which we were the guests. He said that he had always been "hyper" and had been placed on Ritalin when he was a child. He went on to add that the medication was increased over time but never really helped him "do better in school." Finally, when he was a teenager, another doctor saw him and immediately tested his thyroid function. The physician diagnosed hyperthyroidism, a condition in which the gland produces too much hormone, causing fidgetiness. With the proper treatment for this problem, his anxiety and overactivity went away.

We were indebted to this young man for sharing his story on the air. He made our point about the importance of a good physical examination better than we could.

It is important to note that the opposite condition, hypothyroidism (in which the thyroid produces too little hormone), can also present problems. Brad came for testing because his parents and fourth-grade teachers were concerned that he was unable to concentrate. Our initial reaction was that he appeared lethargic and possibly depressed. He was overweight and became easily fatigued.

We discovered that Brad had not been to a pediatrician in a very long time because his family was new to the area. We immediately referred the child to a pediatrician, who determined that Brad was suffering from hypothyroidism. Once the problem was controlled by thyroid medication, the youngster became more upbeat and had greater energy for all kinds of activities, including concentrating in school.

Other symptoms of a thyroid dysfunction include excessive mood swings and irritability. Your doctor can check for other symptoms of a thyroid disorder and can administer any blood tests to monitor thyroid dysfunction, if needed.

Diabetes or Hypoglycemia

Again, while it is rare, it is possible for fluctuations in blood sugar levels to affect concentration and alertness. Zach was a teenage boy referred by his parents for testing because of his poor school performance and problems with attention. Despite a family history of diabetes, his parents had not detected any signs of the disease in their son. After Zach described some of the difficulties he was having, it appeared they were related to when and what he ate. Referral to his family doctor led to the discovery that he was indeed borderline diabetic, and he was put on a therapeutic diet. Later Zach developed a full case of diabetes and required insulin injections. By then everyone understood why his attention level varied throughout the day.

Diabetes is not always the cause of fluctuations in blood sugar. Sometimes the cause is the opposite condition: hypoglycemia. Ellen was a ten-year-old girl who was described as "moody." She became more agitated at certain times of the day, but also became easily fatigued. She was described as having too short an attention span to complete both her morning and afternoon work. In the evenings, her parents complained about her temper and the difficulty they had getting her to complete homework assignments. They said that sometimes her mood seemed to even out after she had a snack. They went to their family physician, who explained that while it was rare, it was possible that Ellen was suffering from hypoglycemia. A glucose tolerance test came back positive. By working with a nutritionist referred by the doctor, Ellen learned how to eat properly to control her condition. Both Ellen's behavior and concentration improved on the new regimen.

In Table 3.3 you will find a list of symptoms of diabetes and hypoglycemia that may serve as a quick reference for you.

Table 3.3
Symptoms of Diabetes and Hypoglycemia

Diabetes
_____ Frequent and increased urination.
_____ New onset of bed-wetting.
_____ Excessive thirst, loss of weight.
_____ Paleness, dark circles under eyes.
_____ Irritability, sweatiness, confusion, extreme hunger.

Hypoglycemia
_____ Brief losses of attention.
_____ Ongoing difficulty with congestion, sleeplessness.
_____ Paleness, lethargy.

Allergies

The media have vigorously promoted the possible link between allergies and attentional deficits. Usually when people consider the link between allergies and ADHD, they automatically think of Dr. Benjamin Feingold. Dr. Feingold's 1975 book *Why Your Child Is Hyperactive* attributed all of the symptoms of attentional deficits and hyperactivity to reactions to certain foods and food additives. As we will discuss in Chapter 11, the Feingold diet was designed to remove all additives from a child's diet. While there were many who became believers in the diet, carefully controlled studies have failed to replicate the improvements Dr. Feingold ascribed to his eating regimen. In fact, further research in this area has also failed to show a conclusive link between elements of the diet and ADHD.

The controversy over food allergies and ADHD does not eliminate the fact that other allergies may influence a child's ability to concentrate and learn. There are a number of children and adults who experience asthma or other respiratory ailments and who have allergic reactions to elements in the environment—all of which can affect concentration. Sometimes the clue to such problems is a pattern in the times of year when difficulties occur. Noting a seasonal pattern in the wheezing, stuffiness, irritated eyes, or other symptoms will help identify possible sources for the problem.

If you are a sufferer, you know how uncomfortable and annoying allergies can be. However, you may not have attributed problems with concentration to this source, nor may you have recognized this problem in yourself or your child. If you suspect that allergies are affecting you or your child in these ways, you should discuss this with your physician.

Unfortunately, the treatments that alleviate closed airways and dry up secretions in the nasal passages sometimes also negatively affect concentration. Even medications that do not cause drowsiness can have side effects that work against concentration and attention by making the person agitated and seem fidgety. If you notice any of these side effects, report them to your physician.

Neurological Disorders

When most people think of seizures, they imagine someone falling on the floor, with eyes rolling back into the head, and becoming unconscious. Another form of seizure activity, petit mal, is much milder and sometimes overlooked.

In general, a petit mal seizure involves a momentary loss of awareness so fleeting that even the person experiencing it may not notice. An onlooker may note some rapid blinking, but it's more likely the person will simply stare briefly into space or seem inattentive. Such behavior could easily be confused with daydreaming. A distinguishing clue to this type of seizure is the person's inability to remember what has happened. However, since the episodes usually occur randomly over time, they often go unreported.

Your doctor should be told about any periods of staring, blinking, and loss of awareness/memory that you or your child experiences. During a physical exam, your physician may look for "soft" neurological signs of a problem, including difficulties with balance, coordination, and muscle tone, by having the individual do some visual tracking exercises or other maneuvers.

Sometimes more testing is needed to rule out any problems. A doctor may send you or your child to a neurologist for an EEG (brain wave test) to rule out other types of neurological problems. Don't panic. Even if petit mal seizure activity is discovered, it often responds well to medication and rarely leads to more serious seizure activity.

STEP 3. RULE OUT PRIMARY EMOTIONAL/PSYCHOLOGICAL PROBLEMS.

A person may have psychological or emotional problems that interfere with attention and concentration, or that leave him feeling so agitated that he seems fidgety or "hyper." Of course, ADHD itself often complicates daily life so much that a person feels many of the same things. So which comes first: the ADHD or emotional problems? A psychologist, a psychiatrist, or another mental health professional can determine whether anxiety, depression, or behavior or thought disorders are causing symptoms that resemble ADHD.

Anxiety

When anyone gets anxious or nervous it is harder to concentrate. Imagine you are waiting for someone you love to arrive at your home. The appointed time passes, and the person doesn't call. As the minutes tick by, you become more concerned. You try to watch a television show or read, but it's difficult. Your mind keeps returning to the question, Where is he or she? It's difficult to think of anything else.

Imagine that you are about to speak in front of a large group of your peers. You have worked hard on your presentation, but it is very impor- tant that you do well. Your heart may race, your body may tense up. You may "block" on an otherwise innocuous question someone asks you and may find it difficult to concentrate.

In both of these situations you may appear anxious as you repeat- edly sit down, stand up, and pace back and forth. To the casual observer you may appear dazed or "out of it." Anxiety makes it difficult to con- centrate.

Adults are often able to express their anxiety in words. Children, however, don't commonly label these feelings. They may not even be aware that anxiety is what they are experiencing. However, an onlooker may notice a child picking and biting at his nails, twirling her hair, twitching, or displaying other "nervous habits." Even without such tell- tale signs, a child may be so anxious that he becomes fidgety and cannot concentrate.

Anxiety can also be caused by other problems. Susan was referred to us because she could not complete a simple task in the classroom. Even drawing a simple picture was difficult. For example, during one of our sessions, we asked her to draw a picture of herself. She made several attempts but erased each one. Finally, she tore a hole in the paper and asked for another piece to begin again. After thirty minutes she reluc- tantly handed over a picture she clearly did not like. Susan was equally displeased with other products—a short story, math problems, her hand- writing—and became more and more distressed over time. She repeat- edly erased her work and checked and rechecked her answers for misspelling, poorly formed letters, and other "mistakes."

Perfectionism like Susan's interferes with her ability to complete a task in a reasonable length of time. More important, it left her never feeling good about her work. Susan's behavior was extreme. Another individual may simply have difficulty getting started on a task or, ironi- cally, may alleviate anxiety by rushing through the job so quickly she can rationalize, "I really didn't try to do my best."

Often people who are perfectionistic are afraid to risk making a mis- take or looking foolish. They may not ask questions or get needed infor- mation for fear of social embarrassment.

In order to determine if anxiety is the cause of either your own or your child's problems, you may need to see a psychologist, a psychiatrist, or another mental health professional. There are a number of standard- ized psychological tests that measure anxiety in different situations, as a basic personality trait or part of a problem like perfectionism. A trained professional will also elicit a complete history and conduct a clinical interview to determine whether anxiety is a primary problem causing inattention, or whether it coexists with ADHD.

Depression

In past decades, depression was hidden until it became so severe that people were labeled as having "nervous breakdowns." In its extreme form, depression can lead to a "shutting down" in which the person withdraws from the outside world.

Even mild depression can disrupt attention and concentration. Many people assume depression means withdrawal and despondency. In fact, though, there are many depressed individuals who go to work and complete their chores daily, without showing any outward signs of depression. Their concentration is interrupted by negative thoughts and feelings, and they worry obsessively about something that has happened or may occur. Their depression may also cause them to become agitated, and this may be misinterpreted as restlessness or fidgetiness. Sleep and appetite may also be affected.

It is only recently that the public has begun to understand that depression can also affect children and adolescents. Sometimes a tragedy predicts its onset, but that is not always the case.

Jeremy was in high school when he was referred to the clinic for attention problems in school. His teachers reported that he spent a lot of time daydreaming in class and often could not answer questions when called on. In our first session, Jeremy said that he never got distracted by others talking or things occurring in the classroom. He also denied daydreaming. When asked what he thought about while in school, he became quiet. After a long pause he began to talk about his parents' divorce and his worries about his mother's financial problems. Recently he'd had trouble sleeping and was tired in school. Other comments he made and his score on an adolescent depression scale indicated that he was in fact depressed.

A number of different psychological tests and procedures are used to assess depression in individuals of different ages. In younger children these frequently take the form of drawings and diagnostic play, as well as standardized parent and teacher questionnaires. For older children and adolescents, questionnaires remain a valuable source of diagnostic information. With adults, there are a variety of standardized tests that assess depression and other emotional factors. These measures, along with skilled clinical judgment, are needed to determine what type of depression, if any, is present and how it is affecting functioning.

Behavior Disorders

A child or adolescent with ADHD may at times become extremely angry and defiant. Sometimes ADHD youth also have a conduct or oppositional defiant disorder.

Conduct disorders and oppositional defiant disorders are distinct diagnoses relating to specific patterns of behavior. They may occur in isolation or in combination with ADHD.

The child with ADHD alone does not seem to be as angry or as oppositional as the child who has both ADHD and a conduct disorder. A child with the oppositional disorder always seeks someone else to blame for what befalls him. In addition, his behavior is often not as spontaneous or impulsive as that of a child with ADHD alone. The ADHD child may display quick angry outbursts; in contrast, there is often an element of planning and conniving in the disruptions and rebellion against authority of the child who has a conduct disorder. Sometimes the behavior of an ADHD child or youth resembles that of a youth with a behavior disorder, but the non-ADHD child with a simple conduct disorder rarely has the restlessness and distractibility associated with ADHD.

To distinguish ADHD and other behavior disorders, or combinations of the two, requires a skilled clinician. Without the correct diagnosis, treatment will be incomplete and ineffective.

Thought Disorders

This rare class of psychological problems may be a disguised cause of concentration problems. Thought disorders may involve hallucinations, wherein the person hears voices that distract him or sees things that are not there. Occasionally a child we are testing pauses almost in mid-sentence as though she were hearing something in the hall. When questioned, she may reveal that she sometimes hears voices that tell her to act in certain ways. Another child may look around the room or stare off into space. He later reports that he saw a "vision." Both of these are unusual cases.

Youngsters and young adults like these may also demonstrate behavioral and psychological symptoms of prepsychotic or psychotic disorders. The flow of their conversation may be hard to follow; their thinking may be illogical, and they may persistently go off on tangents.

Stimulant medication should not be prescribed for people with thought disorders. A different form of treatment requiring other forms of medication may be required. Although we don't want to be alarming, mistaking and treating someone with a thought disorder as having ADHD can lead to the kinds of horror stories reported in the media. Hallucinations and delusions are symptoms of severe psychological disorders that require specific treatment to prevent an individual from possibly hurting himself or others.

The existence of thought disorders is usually detected in a clinical interview conducted by a trained professional. Other tests may be needed to confirm the nature of the thought problems.

STEP 4. DETERMINE IF THERE ARE LEARNING DISABILITIES OR LEARNING DEFICITS.

Often, one of the main reasons children are referred for attention deficit disorder is that they are having trouble staying on-task and completing work in school. While these observed behaviors can be the result of inattention, there are other important reasons why a child might be having such troubles in school and outside of the classroom.

One of the most common discoveries we find in working with children who have severe difficulty completing tasks and succeeding in the classroom is that they have learning disabilities. In the 1980s the term *learning disability* was bandied about almost as often as ADHD is, resulting in confusion about what the term actually means.

Many people think that a learning disability occurs only when an individual sees or writes letters and words backwards. Dyslexia, a well-known learning problem, is only one of many kinds of learning disabilities. Some learning disabilities are less obvious to the observer and remain largely hidden during a child's school career. A learning disability is first defined as a problem in learning that is not the result of poor intelligence or poor teaching. In other words, the individual has average or above-average intelligence but fails to learn despite good instruction.

The second part of the definition of a learning disability relates to the way a person handles information. A learning disability may involve the perception or intake of information, the processing of information, or the expression of information. For example, a visual perception problem interferes with the individual's ability to recognize or discriminate shapes, letters, or words. With a different type of learning disability, another person may have no difficulty recognizing words but may have problems comprehending information or remembering it. Still another individual may not be able to blend the sounds of letters to make words, express himself orally, or spell.

Learning disabilities take many different forms. A child may have difficulty sequencing information or remembering directions that are presented orally. On the other hand, the same child may have no problem with a seemingly more difficult task. Or he may have an easy time with numbers, but a terrible time with letters and words. That's what makes learning disabilities so frustrating for those who have them. You can do one task in one area and have an impossible time with a supposedly "easier" task in another subject.

Not surprisingly, a learning disability can severely block learning. It is important to note that about one third of the children who are legitimately diagnosed ADHD also have other learning disabilities. In addition, 40 percent of the children who have learning disabilities have an attention deficit. Thus, as shown in Figure 3.1, there are quite a number of children who have both a learning disability and an attention deficit disorder. The combination certainly puts a student at a disadvantage in the classroom.

Individuals—both children and adults—with undiagnosed and untreated learning disabilities will go through all kinds of gyrations to hide the problem. They may become great at "covering," as Christopher Lee catalogs so clearly in his book *Faking It.* They are also likely to daydream, leave work uncompleted, seem disorganized, and avoid situations that might expose their weaknesses. In fact, they can look a lot like people with an attention deficit disorder. Once again, the correct diagnosis is crucial: Medication will have no effect on a learning disability.

There are, finally, many children who are simply not achieving in school. For whatever reasons—lapses in attendance, changes of schools, home problems—children sometimes accumulate gaps in knowledge that make it difficult to progress. Once a student gets behind, he often gets frustrated and attempts to hide his deficit. Such deficiencies can strain a normal attention span and make someone look ADHD even though he is not.

If you suspect that you or your child has either a learning disability or learning deficits, a "psychoeducational" evaluation will provide the information you need. A psychologist and/or other learning specialists

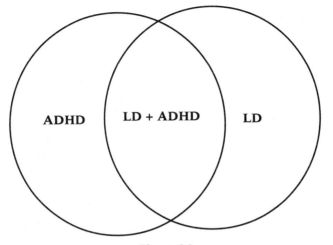

Figure 3.1
The Proportion of Children with Both ADHD and LD

will administer appropriate tests to determine learning potential, information-processing abilities, and academic achievement.

STEP 5. USE THE CRITERIA FOR ADHD.

If you are following the diagnostic trail, by now you have eliminated
medical, psychological, and emotional problems and have identified any
obstacles to learning. Now you are ready to judge whether the diagnostic
criteria for ADHD match the characteristics you or your child displays.

In 1994 the American Psychiatric Association (APA) published the
Fourth Edition of its *Diagnostic and Statistical Manual of Mental Disorders*
(*DSM-IV*), which physicians and psychologists use to identify all kinds of
psychological problems that people may have, ranging from stress and
adjustment problems to more serious disorders. *DSM-IV* divides the disorder known as ADHD into three subtypes.

1. ADHD, Combined Type

The criteria for inattention and hyperactivity listed below in *DSM-IV* must
be present for the past six months.

2. ADHD, Predominantly Inattentive Type

The criteria for inattention but not those for hyperactivity and impulsivity listed below must be met for the past six months.

3. ADHD, Predominantly Hyperactive-Impulsive Type
The criteria for hyperactivity and impulsivity but not inattention must be met for the past six months.

DIAGNOSTIC CRITERIA FOR
ATTENTION-DEFICIT/HYPERACTIVITY DISORDER

A. Either (1) or (2).

(1) six (or more) of the following symptoms of inattention have persisted for at least six months to a degree that is maladaptive and inconsistent with developmental level:

Inattention
(a) often fails to give close attention to details or makes careless mistakes in schoolwork, work, or other activities
(b) often has difficulties sustaining attention in tasks or play activities
(c) often does not seem to listen when spoken to directly
(d) often does not follow through on instructions and fails to finish schoolwork, chores, or duties in the workplace (not due to oppositional behavior or failure to understand instructions).
(e) often has difficulty organizing tasks and activities
(f) often avoids, dislikes, or is reluctant to engage in tasks that require sustained mental effort (such as schoolwork or homework)
(g) often loses things necessary for tasks or activities (e.g., toys, school assignments, pencils, books, or tools)
(h) is often easily distracted by extraneous stimuli
(i) is often forgetful in daily activities

(2) six (or more) of the following symptoms of hyperactivity-impulsivity have persisted for at least six months to a degree that is maladaptive and inconsistent with developmental level:

Hyperactivity
(a) often fidgets with hands or feet or squirms in seat
(b) often leaves seat in classroom or in other situations in which remaining seated is expected
(c) often runs about or climbs excessively in situations in which it is inappropriate (in adolescents or adults, may be limited to subjective feelings of restlessness)
(d) often has difficulty playing or engaging in leisure activities quietly

(e) is often "on the go" or often acts as if "driven by a motor"

(f) often talks excessively

Impulsivity

(g) often blurts out answers before questions have been completed

(h) often has difficulty awaiting turn

(i) often interrupts or intrudes on others (e.g., butts into conversations or games)

B. Some hyperactive-impulsive or inattentive symptoms that caused impairment were present before age seven.

C. Some impairment from the symptoms is present in two or more settings (e.g., at school, at work, or at home).

D. There must be clear evidence of clinically significant impairment in social, academic, or occupational functioning.

E. The symptoms do not occur exclusively during the course of pervasive developmental disorder, schizophrenia, or other psychotic disorders, and are not better accounted for by another mental disorder (e.g., mood disorder, anxiety disorder, dissociative disorder, or personality disorder).

Adapted from *DSM-IV*, Washington, D.C.: American Psychiatric Association, 1994, pp. 83–85.

While a trained professional must make the diagnosis of ADHD, your understanding of the diagnostic criteria is an important first step for you.

STEP 6. GET RATINGS/OBSERVATIONS FROM AS MANY SETTINGS AS POSSIBLE.

ADHD may manifest itself in distinct ways in different settings and at different times. The best way to accurately measure the various aspects of ADHD is to gather observations from as many different settings as possible.

The easiest way to gather such information is through rating scales and overt measures of distractibility and attention. A rating scale is an objective way for an observer—perhaps a teacher, coworker, or friend who knows you or your child—to communicate what he or she has seen over time. Those comments can be compared with observations about many other adults or children to determine whether a particular behavior is common or more unusual, or whether a pattern of behavior is indicative of a particular kind of problem.

There are a number of rating scales that can be used for children and adolescents. Because each *instrument,* as these scales are called, may measure different factors, we suggest using two instruments. For children, it is also important to get ratings not only from present teachers but also when possible from previous teachers. This information will provide a picture of your child's behavior in various situations, over time, as it is judged by a number of people who have a great deal of experience with children. Add your own ratings of your child's behavior and you will have a fuller understanding of your child's activity level and attention at home and school.

Parent Ratings for Children and Adolescents
Conners Parent Rating Scales (CPRS)

Dr. C. Keith Conners developed three different versions of the CPRS starting in 1970. The original has ninety-three questions and is the most extensive. It yields a number of emotional and behavioral factors in addition to hyperactivity-immaturity. A revised version published in 1978 has forty-eight questions with fewer items related to anxiety and other internal problems, but still gives valid measures of conduct problems and hyperactivity. These rating scales are easy to score and are among the most widely used by pediatricians, psychologists, and psychiatrists. The third Conners rating form is a ten-item abbreviated version to be used to help monitor medication effects once a diagnosis has been made.

The Child Behavior Checklist (CBCL)

The CBCL was developed by Drs. Achenbach and Edelbrock in 1983. It has two parts. The first part, with twenty questions, gives a social competence score in activities and school. The remaining 118 questions yield scores for:

1. Internalizing factors such as anxiety, withdrawal, and psychosomatic complaints.
2. Externalizing factors such as aggression and delinquency.
3. Attentional, thought, and social problems.

The comprehensive nature of this instrument gives a professional information needed to assess other problems that may mimic ADHD, as well as attentional factors.

Attention-Deficit/Hyperactivity Disorder Test (ADHDT)

The ADHDT is a new rating scale based on *DSM-IV* criteria that can be used to identify individuals, between three and twenty-three years of age, who are ADHD. The scale has thirty-six items and three subtests: hyperactivity, impulsivity, and inattention. One form of the ADHDT (unlike other rating scales) may be completed by teachers, parents, and others who know the individual. The norms collected in 1993 and 1994 on a national sample of twelve hundred people diagnosed with ADHD are presented separately for males and females.

Teacher Ratings for Children and Adolescents
Conners Teacher Rating Scale (CTRS)

There are several versions of the CTRS. The original had thirty-nine items. The revised version has twenty-eight, and there is also an abbreviated version. The thirty-nine-item version gives the most factors, including hyperactivity as well as conduct problems, emotional-overindulgent, anxious-passive, asocial, and daydreaming/inattention. This instrument provides the doctor with much-needed information to help make a diagnosis. The CTRS has been shown to be accurate in measuring medication effects.

Children's Behavior Checklist—Teacher's Report Form (CBCL-TRF)

This checklist is similar to the parent's CBCL. However, in the teacher's version the first part of the test gives a measure of how the child is adapting in the classroom. The second section again provides measures of internal problems, external conduct problems, and attentional problems.

ADD-H Comprehensive Teacher Rating Scale (ACTeRS)

The chief use of this rating scale is found in its ability to discriminate children who are ADHD from those with learning disabilities, and those who have an attention deficit with and without hyperactivity. The teacher rating scale has twenty-four items and is appropriate for children from five to twelve years old.

Continuous-Performance Tasks for Children, Adolescents, and Adults

A number of clinical and laboratory tasks have been developed to measure various aspects of attention. *Continuous-performance tasks* (CPT) are tests of vigilance or attention span. Although there are many ways to do this, the most popular require the individual to observe a screen while numbers or letters are flashed at a rapid pace. The individual is told to press a button when a target, a particular stimulus, or a sequence of stimuli appears on the screen. The number of correct responses, the number of target items missed, and the number of items misidentified as the target form the basis of the score.

Computerized measures of attention should never be used in isolation to diagnose ADHD. Recent studies by Dr. Russell Barkley have shown that the incidence of false negatives on these tests can be high. In these cases a person may do well on a continuous-performance task and still suffer from ADHD. However, approximately 90 percent of the children who obtain an abnormal score are ADHD.

The Gordon Diagnostic System

The Gordon Diagnostic System is a solid-state, childproof, computerized device that is designed to measure a child's attention. During a nine-minute vigilance task, the child must press a button each time a particular target appears on a screen. The Gordon also includes two other nine-minute tasks that measure impulsivity and distractibility.

The Test of Variables of Attention (TOVA)

The TOVA is another visual continuous-performance task that is programmed for use with IBM compatibles, Apple, and Macintosh computers. Developed by Dr. Lawrence Greenberg at the University of Minnesota, this continuous-performance task is nonlanguage-based to discriminate ADHD from learning disabilities. The task lasts for 11.5 minutes for four- and five-year-olds and 22.5 minutes for individuals from six to eighty years of age.

Employing a Trained Observer

You may also find it helpful and interesting to have a trained observer whom your child does not know do a classroom observation. It may supply significant, valuable details about your child's behavior, the behavior of other children in the classroom, how the teacher runs her classroom, and the types of experiences provided. For example, you may be surprised to learn that your child is one of many students who are out of their seats and unable to attend, because the classroom is generally "out of control." Or you may find that the observer confirms the ratings already collected.

Rating Scales for Adults

At present, there are no standardized rating instruments for adult ADHD, but several diagnostic tools may prove helpful. The above-mentioned TOVA may be helpful when learning disabilities are suspected. Dr. Paul Wender and colleagues developed the Utah Criteria for the Diagnosis of ADD Residual Type. *DSM-IV* describes the cause of ADHD in adults. And Dr. Russell Barkley has developed the most detailed structured interview for ADHD. He also gets ratings not only from the client but also from the spouse and even from parents when possible.

To obtain an accurate adult diagnosis of ADHD, be sure the professional you are working with uses a detailed approach to diagnosis, such as the one developed by Dr. Barkley.

STEP 7. MAKING THE DIAGNOSIS AND DETERMINING A TREATMENT PLAN.

Through the years you have probably felt that your behavior or your child's was a puzzlement. Now you have the pieces of the puzzle. If they fit into the pattern described by *DSM-IV*, then a diagnosis of attention deficit hyperactivity disorder can be made.

It's important to keep in mind that a diagnosis is a starting point, not an end. From this point, you should be able to a gain better understanding of your behavior or your child's. You will be more able to predict those situations that may be difficult, and you will gain a new respect for the rediscovered strengths you may have forgotten. Most important, you can begin a treatment plan that can help you or your child get back on the road to success.

As we have said many times, *medication should never be the sole treatment for ADHD*. An effective treatment plan for ADHD may include medication and, at various times, behavioral interventions at home and school, social-skills training, individual and family therapy, specialized tutoring, and other elements that you or your child needs to learn to cope.

The Diagnostic Checklist presented in Table 3.4 may be used as a guide as you work through the diagnostic steps and record the information you gather about yourself or your child. Keep in mind that the Diagnostic Checklist and the information presented in this chapter cannot serve as a substitute for a diagnosis made by a trained professional.

Table 3.4

Diagnostic Checklist

Directions: Working with a physician, a psychologist, and other professionals, use the following checklist to be sure you have eliminated any problems that may strain your child's or your own attention, concentration, and impulse control. Also keep a record of other pertinent information that will help determine treatment for ADHD.

1. Medical Problems That Can Mimic ADHD
_____ Vision Checked
_____ Hearing Screened
_____ Thyroid Function Normal
_____ Diabetes and Hypoglycemia Eliminated

2. Emotional Problems That Can Interfere with Concentration
_____ Anxiety Disorders
_____ Depression/Mood Disorders
_____ Personality Disorders
_____ Thought Disorders (including hallucinations)

3. Get two different rating forms filled out by parents and teachers (see pages 47–51 for suggested rating instruments). Record the name of the rating instruments and whether the ratings were significant.

	Rating Scale	Rating 1	Rating 2
Father			
Mother			
Teacher 1			
Teacher 2			
Teacher 3			

For adults, use a structured interview and observations or ratings from parents and spouse. See page 51 for more details.

4. Record notes from classroom observations.
Date of Observation: _____
Observer: _____

Significant Observations: _____
_____
_____
_____
_____

5. Have a professional conduct a psycoeducational evaluation. The form below shows the kinds of information he/she will collect.

Evaluation by _____		**Date** _____		
LEARNING POTENTIAL	**SUPERIOR**	**ABOVE AVERAGE**	**AVERAGE**	**BELOW AVERAGE**
ACHIEVEMENT LEVEL	**Above Grade**		**On Grade**	**Below Grade**
Math				
Language Arts				
Spelling				
Written Expression				
Reading				
Learning Disabilites or Areas of Difficulty				
Learning Gaps				

6. Use the following snap checklist based on *DSM-IV* to determine if child or adult characteristics meet ADHD criteria.

Check those symptoms that describe you or your child.

Inattention

_____ 1. Often fails to give close attention to details or makes careless mistakes in schoolwork, work, or other activities.

_____ 2. Often has difficulty sustaining attention in tasks or play activities.

_____ 3. Often does not seem to listen when spoken to directly.

_____ 4. Often does not follow through on instructions and fails to finish schoolwork, chores, or duties in the workplace.

_____ 5. Often has difficulty organizing tasks and activities.

_____ 6. Often avoids, dislikes, or is reluctant to engage in tasks that require sustained mental effort, such as schoolwork or homework.

_____ 7. Often loses things necessary for tasks or activities, such as toys, school assignments, pencils, books, or tools.

_____ 8. Is often easily distracted by extraneous stimuli.

_____ 9. Is often forgetful in daily activities.

Hyperactivity-Impulsivity

_____ 1. Often fidgets with hands or feet or squirms in seat.

_____ 2. Often leaves seat in classroom or in other situations in which remaining seated is expected.

_____ 3. Often runs about or climbs excessively in situations in which it is inappropriate (in adolescents or adults, may be limited to subjective feelings of restlessness).

_____ 4. Often has difficulty playing or engaging in leisure activities quietly.

_____ 5. Is often "on the go" or often acts as if "driven by a motor."

_____ 6. Often talks excessively.

_____ 7. Often blurts out answers before questions have been completed.

_____ 8. Often has difficulty awaiting turn.

_____ 9. Often interrupts or intrudes on others (e.g., butts into conversations or games).

Did you check six or more characteristics under Inattention?

Did you check six or more characteristics under Hyperactivity-Impulsivity?

Have you made sure these characteristics are not due to developmental, medical, or psychological problems?

Have these characteristics existed for the past six months or more?

Are they more pronounced than in same-age peers?

Do they cause some impairment in two or more settings?

A FINAL WORD ON DIAGNOSIS

As you read through the rest of the book, use the following form to make notes as to the kinds of treatment that may be appropriate to your situation. If you or your child meets the criteria for ADHD, the following chart will help you plan and consider the elements of treatment that may be appropriate.

Table 3.5

Planning and Coordinating Treatment for ADHD

	ADHD IMPULSIVE	ADHD INATTENTIVE	LEARNING DISABILITIES	SOCIAL PROBLEMS	EMOTIONAL PROBLEMS	CONDUCT DISORDER
Environmental Engineering						
Behavior Therapy						
Educational Therapy						
Social Skills						
Individual Therapy						
Family Therapy						
Parent Training						

4

WHAT TO TRY BEFORE YOU TRY MEDICATION

Alternatives at School, Home, and Work

As an adult with ADHD, you may be eager to discover what effects medication has on your problems, but we have never met a parent who was as anxious to use medication to improve his or her child's attention, concentration, impulsivity, or hyperactivity. Every parent we meet wants to know if there's an alternative approach they can try first. The answer is often yes. There are a number of options that you may try before turning to medication. If you eventually decide to use medication, you should remember that each of these alternatives may be even more effective when used in conjunction with medication.

MAINSTREAM INTERVENTIONS THAT CAN MAKE A DIFFERENCE

Most people associate the term *alternative medicine* with "off the beaten path," unproven, or unscientific remedies. In this case, "alternative" interventions are very much *on the beaten path* and in the mainstream of good practice. In fact, it is erroneous and misleading to consider these treatments alternative simply because they do not involve medication. They are first and foremost effective educational and psychological practices that may make it possible for you or your child to function successfully without medication. If you choose to try medication at some point, the research literature has provided evidence that these interventions in combination with medication often work better than either approach alone. The suggested treatments in this chapter may make it possible for you to use less medication, for less of the day, and perhaps, in time, to eliminate medication altogether.

The key element in all of these alternative treatments is the element of *change:* in one's environment, in the way tasks are presented, and in one's behavior. There are numerous reasons why a particular change could make a major difference in your situation. These factors vary with the demands of the learning or work environment, the severity of the ADHD, and other individual traits.

Alternative treatments for ADHD that may have been or continue to be unproven, controversial, or unconventional are fully presented in Chapter 11, "Alternative Treatments: Fads, Fallacies, and Facts." Here we discuss proven practices that can be adapted to your situation. These interventions center on three elements of change:

1. Making changes at home, at school, or in the work environment to improve functioning.
2. Altering the task to improve production.
3. Adopting behavioral interventions that help the individual modify ADHD behavior patterns.

These three elements of change have relevancy both for the ADHD student at school and home, and for the ADHD adult in a work environment. The first part of this discussion pertains to children and adolescents. Later on in the chapter we focus on nonmedical interventions specifically for adults.

ENVIRONMENTAL MODIFICATIONS THAT HELP PRODUCTIVITY

Changing behavior is difficult. However, modifying the immediate environment will often bring about a positive behavior and a better outcome. Before you try changing your child or yourself, you may be able to alter the school, work, or living situation to gain the same results. These "environmental interventions" involve changes in where, with whom, when, and how you work, study, and operate at home.

AT SCHOOL

Change Where Your Child Sits in the Classroom

The simple act of switching where your child sits in the classroom may have a dramatic effect on concentration and behavior. That's not as amazing as it sounds. For years, teachers have relocated children in the classroom, away from a particular classmate, or closer to the teacher, to control disruptive behavior. Several studies and a great deal of teacher experience indicate that classroom seating has an impact on children's proneness to pay attention. This is especially true of ADHD youth.

In general, seating students at tables or in circles is great for social interactions and small group discussion, but not very good for independent work. Distractions and off-task behavior increase in such a setting. On the other hand, sitting in rows leads to increased seat work, but it's not great when the teacher begins lecturing. Circle seating may help students pay attention to lectures and oral discussions, but may be less effective for independent tasks.

Choose a Place Based on the Traffic Flow.

For some children, the front desk of the row closest to the teacher's desk is the optimum seat in the classroom. However, it could backfire horribly for your child if the teacher's desk is a center of activity and more distracting than his present location. On the other hand, if your child is one who must know what all his friends are doing, then sitting at the front of the classroom will only give him a super crick in the neck. In that case, he would probably be better off sitting in the back of the room away from the action but where he can peruse the situation and then get back to work.

Choose a Location Free of Intermittent Noises, Sights, and Changing Scenery.

For similar reasons, it's usually not a good idea to seat an ADHD child near the pencil sharpener, an exterior door, a busy work station, or any other frequently trafficked location. The constant buzz of activity is bound to distract him. Also avoid any location with changing scenery, such as a window or door, or anyplace students initiate individual or group work.

Consider the Ramifications of Isolation.

It's a common classroom practice to move a disruptive child's desk away from everyone else. Less disruptive but easily distracted students are also sometimes separated from their distractions by isolating their desks.

Teachers have created shields and built carrels out of cardboard boxes and refrigerator crates to screen visual distractions from the student's view. Some schools have gone to the additional expense of partitioning the special classroom into cubicles. Unfortunately, the source of the greatest distraction for many ADHD students emanates from the mind and body, so while these efforts may block external visual distractors, they cannot prevent ADHD students from daydreaming, doodling, and doing whatever else takes them off-task. In addition, isolation can have the unfortunate side effect of making a child whose self-esteem is already slipping feel ostracized.

Use Trial and Error to Find the Least Distracting Location in the Classroom.

There is no one place in a classroom that is the best for an ADHD child. Finding the least distracting position for your child in each particular classroom is a process of trial and error that you will have to repeat for each teacher's style of presentation, each classroom's size and layout, and the demands of each class's subject matter.

Everyone involved—you, your child, and the teacher—must be open to experimenting to find the best seat. Once you have discovered what works best for your child in that class, you can communicate the information to other teachers.

As your child moves into the intermediate and upper grades, and becomes more astute about his own learning style, he should be encouraged to become his own best advocate. Adolescents need and prefer to speak for themselves. Furthermore, a teacher is more likely to listen to a student who presents the facts of her case. Even more important, as your student grows older this will be valuable information she can put to use when she must choose her own seat in college classrooms or arrange her environment at work.

Change School Routines
Vary the Class Schedule.

Although an elementary student has little control over the day's schedule, any information you can gather about when your student works best is valuable.

Sometimes in high school, the school counselor and registrar will work with you to schedule courses that require high concentration at a time of day that is best for your student. One high school student we worked with did very poorly in history when it was scheduled as the last class of the day. In his senior year, however, his grades improved markedly, without medication. The simple solution: scheduling history for right after lunch, when he wasn't so fatigued and had just eaten.

Of course, knowing his best time of day will be a great asset as your youngster approaches college. There he may have more flexibility in scheduling classes and more leeway in arranging to take exams during his peak concentration times. Knowing when to schedule classes can be the determining factor in success or failure for an ADHD student.

Identify a Study Buddy.

Pairing an ADHD student with a good role model who stays on-task can promote good work habits at school and at home. Such role models are less distracting and less likely to be distractible. In addition, this student can serve as a "study buddy" to the ADHD student. Without distracting too many other students, your child can verify homework assignments before leaving for home. Depending on how the pairing is planned, a study buddy can prompt the ADHD student to take home books and remind her about upcoming tests. From home, the ADHD student can phone her study buddy to verify assignments and ask questions. Peer tutoring can also be a valuable learning tool for students of all ages.

As the ADHD student grows, she can learn to take positive advantage of her classmates. For example, many ADHD students or students with learning disabilities find it difficult to take good lecture notes; they might borrow notes from another student. An ADHD student might opt to visit the library with friends who are good study partners rather than those who prefer to spend that time socializing.

Change Classrooms or School

Sometimes the match between a student and a teacher or a school doesn't work. Occasionally personalities clash, but in the case of ADHD students, the teacher's teaching style, the classroom arrangement, structure of the day, the school's philosophy and expectations, or the curriculum itself may prevent the match from working. On rare occasions, a child has been so pigeonholed that changing perceptions of him and giving a "new start" would be impossible in the old setting. In addition, by placing the student in a smaller classroom, in a specialized setting, or with a teacher who is skillful at adapting subject matter and materials to the needs of your child, you may be able to avoid medication.

Consider Instructional Patterns.

From year to year and teacher to teacher, you are likely to have received varying reports about your child. You may have even thought sometimes that two teachers were talking about two different children. The fact is that various classroom characteristics and teacher traits influence your child's behavior every day. This is more than simply a matter of the location of his seat: The structure of the classroom, the instructional schedule, and the teacher's style may have a major impact on your child's classroom behavior.

Teachers have different teaching styles; children different learning styles. Each comes into play when you make a match between a student and a classroom or teacher. The best seat in the classroom for your child is likely to change from subject to subject and from teacher to teacher. The teacher's instructional style and the type of tasks will influence where the best seat might be. Some teachers spend most of their time instructing a large group; others break their classes into small groups for most instruction. For some, individualizing instruction is the norm; others provide a number of tasks to meet the same goal, and the students pick and choose their own instruction. In still other classrooms, every student is expected to complete the same set of exercises each day.

Almost any classroom can be made to work for your student, *if* the teacher is willing to make adjustments. We have seen ADHD students who were able to function well seated at small tables as long as the other students at the table were on-task most of the time. Many ADHD students work better in classrooms where the assignments are clearly structured but the student has some flexibility of movement. For example, in a classroom with centers, as long as the student knows exactly what he needs to accomplish, he may prefer being able to move from center to center.

Arrange for Regular Feedback from the Teacher.

Most ADHD students need structure and thrive on frequent feedback from the teacher. The students need to know what is expected of them and have the tasks presented in a clear sequence. However, if they are given too many tasks to complete, they fall apart. Recognizing how a teacher's instructional style and teaching pattern will work for your child is important.

Joanie's experience is a good example. At 8:00 A.M., when Joanie entered her fourth-grade classroom, the morning assignments were written on the board. Most students looked to the board for their instructions, but Joanie's teacher adapted the routine for her. Attached to a folder on her desk, Joanie found a short checklist of morning work. She didn't need to look to the board or copy work. In addition, inside the folder were two work sheets. When she completed the work sheets, she crossed them off her list and turned to the next assigned task. Her teacher supervised her progress in between instructing small groups of students. This pattern worked for Joanie.

Consider the Layout of the Classroom.

Great instruction can be given anywhere, but the configuration of the classroom does influence the way students function and feel in the setting. Large open classrooms were designed to provide space for many groups of students to work simultaneously with several teachers in a variety of ways. Open classrooms are meant to be busy spaces filled with the noise of learning. Physically, there is sometimes little to soften the noise or impede the view. Such large areas can be very distracting for an ADHD student. It is often surprising to find how much an ADHD student's behavior can change when he is switched from a more "open classroom," or "pod," to a self-contained space housing a more traditional, structured classroom.

Smaller Student-Teacher Ratios Work Better.

The number of students in a classroom is crucial. Often an ADHD student will perform much better in a smaller class. In fact, we have noted that sometimes a student who required medication in a larger classroom may be able to function off medication or with less medication in a smaller setting.

Although most public schools have defined student-teacher ratios, it is sometimes possible to find a smaller class size within a public school setting. If not, there may be a larger class that operates like one with few students if the teacher spends a large portion of the day instructing small groups. This is especially true if there is an assistant teacher assigned to the classroom. The downside of this pattern may be that the student is left to work independently for part of the day and that time must be well structured.

Consider the Teacher's Expectations.

Teachers come in all shapes and sizes. They also vary in the expectations they have about behavior. Your child is likely to respond best to a very positive but firm teacher who defines her behavioral expectations very clearly and sticks to them. Because they are often disorganized and somewhat erratic in their behavior, ADHD children often perform better for a well-organized and well-structured teacher who is knowledgeable about ADHD. An overly permissive teacher is not the best choice, but neither is one who is too rigid or strict. In the latter case, the child can end up a constant source of irritation to the teacher so that they are always butting heads.

Although few principals routinely welcome parents' requests for teachers, we have found that if you discuss the "kind of teacher" and environment in which your child performs best, the suggestions may be heeded. In addition, if you find the right type of teacher for your child one year, often that teacher can become an advocate for your child and work behind the scenes to select an appropriate teacher for the next term.

A Specialized Private School May Provide the Best Setting for an ADHD Child.

There are times when a private school is the best solution for a child's needs. Smaller class size, two teachers in a classroom, specialized teaching, the presence of computers, or other specific components may make the setting a better match for your child.

> After eight-year-old **KAREN** was diagnosed ADHD, her parents decided to place their daughter in a specialized school, with a smaller, very structured classroom headed by a teacher with specialized training. In the new setting, Karen thrived. Assignments were tailored to her academic needs, and a point system motivated her to complete more classwork. Her on-task behavior increased threefold. Since she was not singled out continually for being disruptive, her self-image improved. In this setting, Karen did not need to take medication to be able to manage many of the symptoms of ADHD.

Some ADHD students have attentional difficulties and behavioral habits that make it difficult for them to function in a traditional classroom. Many children who have both learning disabilities and ADHD need not only smaller classes but specialized instruction for part or all of the school day. If this is your child's situation, you may not be able to tell whether or not she will need medication until she receives appropriate instruction or specialized help.

First, explore the options available within your home school. Request a special meeting called a *staffing* to qualify your ADHD student for special programming and/or placement in special classes for ADHD students. The Department of Education's Office of Special Education and Rehabilitative Services issued a memorandum on September 16, 1991, confirming that ADHD is within the scope of the Individuals with Disabilities Education Act of 1975. Accordingly, ADHD must be considered a disability for which public schools must make accommodations and offer special services. If your child does not have a learning disability, the category called Other Health Impaired (OHI) is the proper classification for special help.

In general, we have found teachers and faculties very willing to work with parents to implement practical changes that can make a world of difference to the ADHD child. However, if you discover your child is unable to succeed in the regular classroom, investigate other educational options either within that school or in other facilities. Sometimes a child attending a smaller, specialized school for a year or two can learn self-control skills and study habits for a successful transition back to the home school in the future.

AT HOME

Working at home is difficult for many people, and homework often becomes a major battleground for parents and ADHD children. Assignments that, according to the teacher, should take only minutes could require hours for the ADHD child to complete or could never get done.

Find the Right Homework Location.

A key element of successful homework completion for any child is having the right spot in which to do it. Each student should have a designated homework location with a desk or table, good lighting, a comfortable chair, and the appropriate materials. Where that location is depends on the child.

Most ADHD children require supervision until they learn to manage their own time and work effort, yet few parents have the luxury of doing only one thing at a time. You may have provided the perfect work space, with a great desk and chair and all the right supplies, but unless your child is able to function independently or you can spend time with him, the "perfect" spot may not be the best place. Initially, you may discover that the kitchen table, despite the movement and activities of your preparing dinner, offers the perfect locale for you to supervise homework. Since that spot is also likely to be away from the video games, the computer, and other favorite pastimes, your child will have fewer distractions to ignore.

Time It Right.

Timing is everything. Some of us are morning people; some are not. Some people like to get the work done before they play; others like to take breaks. If your child is ADHD, then timing takes on added significance. To determine what is the best time of day to concentrate, vary her schedule and note the effects.

After being in school all day, many ADHD students find it very difficult to do homework immediately after school. They want and sometimes need to play outdoors or to take a break before returning to work. However, many parents of ADHD students are convinced that unless their youngster does his homework first, it never gets done. Still others find that their youngster performs best when the work is completed in small segments separated by breaks. Again, find the study schedule that works best for your child through trial and error.

CHANGING THE TASK TO INCREASE PRODUCTIVITY

Productivity can be increased by altering the way in which assignments are given, what they look like, and how they are done. ADHD students are often overwhelmed and frustrated by the sheer amount of work that piles up on their desks. Learning to manage the workload takes time.

ALTER THE WAY ASSIGNMENTS ARE GIVEN

Restructuring assignments until youngsters are able to manage their time can have positive effects on performance. We have found teachers who are willing to adjust the kind and amount of assignments they give.

Give Only One Assignment at a Time.
ADHD students have trouble prioritizing tasks and estimating the amount of time each task will take. If they are given a number of tasks at once, they are likely to misplace pages and to become overwhelmed and frustrated. In the classroom, teachers can maximize the ADHD student's output by dispensing assignments one at a time.

Our experiences with Taylor proved this. When his teacher handed out work sheets to complete, or if he saw a number of sentences on the board to copy, seven-year-old Taylor would simply put his head down on his desk. As his classmates got to work, he would play with toys in his pocket, walk around, and generally avoid facing the work. When his teacher began to hand him one assignment at a time, he began work at a reasonable pace. As he finished each task, he put the sheets in the "completed work" bin and got the next assignment from the teacher. It took a little more effort on the teacher's part, but required less time than it took to deal with his previous disruptions.

Help the Student Estimate How Long a Task Will Take.
Few ADHD students have any idea how long a task will take. Most of the time they completely exaggerate the amount of time they will need. The result is that they immediately get frustrated. Helping such a student learn to gauge how long a job will take will alleviate a lot of her fear and frustration.

To teach this skill, Jackie's sixth-grade teacher continued to give him one or two assignments at a time, but she had him look over each assignment and estimate how long it would take to complete. He wrote the minutes on the back of the assignment. When he began a task, he wrote the starting time in the left top corner of the first page. When he completed the work, he jotted down the end time, and determined how long it took him to finish the assignment. Over the year his estimates improved greatly.

Vary Tasks; Break Assignments into Smaller Parts.
For many ADHD children, even one assignment may be too long for them to complete in one sitting. This is probably the prime reason why children and adults with ADHD are labeled as having a "short attention span."

An effective way to overcome this problem is to divide assignments into smaller segments or parts. A child who cannot complete two pages of math problems at one sitting may be able to do one page before getting distracted or daydreaming. If a page is too much, the assignment may have to be further broken down into half-pages. Often, using a top sheet to cover part of a page is a helpful trick. The reinforcement of seeing each part of a task completed gives the student incentive to continue the effort.

Varying the kind of assignment is also effective. Particularly difficult tasks may be interspersed between easier assignments. You may find that certain subjects require more breaks, or that the task must be divided into smaller segments.

Talk with the teacher about using this technique to improve your child's performance and on-task behavior. You may also apply the same procedure at home. Before beginning homework, help your student divide each subject's work into manageable parts. Have him use a timer to see how long he can concentrate on a particular task before his concentration wanes. For example, your student may be able to work on math problems for fifteen minutes at a sitting without getting distracted or off-task. He may be able to read and underline new material for twenty minutes. Using these time frames, help your child estimate the work time and break assignments into units that fit these parameters.

Measuring time and work in this manner is a skill that may help your youngster improve his attention and concentration for homework. As your student becomes more adept, the time limits may increase.

Improve Attention to Directions.
Following directions can be particularly troublesome to ADHD students. Either their minds are elsewhere when the instructions are stated, or they overlook details in the written directions. They often get into trouble for not following directions or may do a task completely wrong because they misread the instructions. It is not uncommon to find that an ADHD student has done only part of a page, has completed all the problems on a page when only the even-numbered problems were assigned, or has undertaken the wrong task altogether.

There are several methods of avoiding these mistakes. For example, an ADHD child should adopt the habit of looking you or the teacher in the eye when oral directions are being given, and then repeating the directions before beginning the task. For printed instructions, have the student underline or circle key words in written directions before beginning a task, or orally verify the instructions with a study buddy. As he works through the task, it is helpful for a student to circle the number for each math problem and to make a check mark next to each completed sentence or problem. After completing a page, have the student put his initials on each page he reviewed for errors or put a dot under each math problem he double-checked.

Alter or Reduce the Written Workload.

Sometimes it is not the task that gets in the way of performance, but the manner of presentation. For many ADHD students, fine motor skills present a problem. The moment they are asked to write something, they freeze. Copying board work, writing full sentences, and filling in small spaces on dittos and in workbooks are an immediate turnoff. If this situation sounds familiar, discuss with your child's teachers ways to modify and reduce the written workload. Instead of having the student copy an assignment from the board, ask the teacher to permit your child to use the original, or allow her to copy key words. Similarly, she may be able to write responses without copying the question itself. Whenever possible, allow the student to demonstrate knowledge by giving oral reports.

Your child is likely to find the computer a very able assistant. The manipulation of computer keys is easier for the child, and the computer itself holds a built-in fascination for many ADHD youths. A number of ADHD students whom we have worked with have even taken laptop computers into the classroom. Some schools permit students to complete the essay parts of exams in the computer center, after writing an outline of their answer in the classroom. Also try using computers to help students not only complete homework but practice new skills such as learning math facts.

You may find a huge change in attitude and productivity simply by altering the manner in which the child must complete the work. For one such child, using the computer made all the difference. It took a great deal of effort for Benjamin to form letters in manuscript or cursive. In addition, his teachers complained about illegibility. Whenever he was presented with a written assignment, it took Ben forever, and his output was minimal. Once he learned to keyboard, he preferred to do all his homework on the computer. His teachers allowed him to go to the computer lab at school to write stories and reports. On other assignments, once he could show he understood the concept or principle, his teachers allowed him to record simple answers.

BEHAVIORAL INTERVENTIONS THAT
ENHANCE POSITIVE RESPONSES

Managing the environment alone, however, will not always bring about the desired changes in behavior. ADHD has been called a deficit in "rule-governed" behavior, because often these children simply don't react to the consequences of their actions in the same way that others do. In addition, they have difficulty inhibiting responses, so they act impulsively, flit from task to task, or respond inappropriately. By strengthening or changing the consequences that follow these actions, you can sometimes help the ADHD youngster to learn to respond more like his peers.

USE SYSTEMATIC PRAISE AND IGNORING

A combination of praising on-task and other appropriate behaviors while ignoring specific inappropriate behaviors may lead to overall improvement in conduct. Sometimes parents and even teachers will tell us they are occasionally afraid to comment when an ADHD child is quiet or working on a task. It is the old "let sleeping dogs lie" syndrome. The adults become fearful that their actions will interrupt the child or cause him to seek negative attention. In fact, however, there are ways to offer positive reinforcement that will not undermine your efforts.

Make Specific, Brief, but Frequent Positive Comments.
If you practice giving frequent, brief comments while systematically ignoring negative, attention-getting behaviors, you can build up positive behaviors.

Begin by standing close to the youngster. Depending on the child's age and personality, you may want to be more or less private in giving praise. Your praise must be specific and immediate: Tell the child what he is doing right.

Praise Observable Behavior.
In each instance, praise actual observable behavior. For example, a teacher might comment, "I like the way you are working on your math problems without even looking up!" Or you might say to your child as she works on her homework, "You have been sitting so quietly while you have been doing your homework for the last ten minutes." Stay away from making statements that praise personality, and avoid global

compliments like, "You are a good girl." These type of comments don't tell the youngster what she is doing right so that she can repeat it. In addition, such comments can backfire over time. Your child may somehow assume he must be "good" all the time. Since that's an impossible accomplishment, he may be reluctant to try.

Ignore Negative Attention-Getting Behaviors.

When any child begins to engage in inappropriate behaviors, especially when they are negative attention-getting, ignoring can be effective. This is also true for ADHD children. When you ignore a behavior, you must remove your complete attention. Look away from the child. Even a brief glance is sometimes enough reinforcement to keep a behavior going. You or the teacher may find that you are best able to ignore the behavior if you move yourself to another location. Don't be surprised if, when you use systematic ignoring, your child's behavior deteriorates at first. As long as your child is attempting to provoke your attention with behaviors that can cause no harm to himself or others, ignore them. If the child engages in other behaviors that you cannot ignore, you will have to use one of the other techniques discussed below. Whenever your child stops the negative behavior and displays any positive behavior, immediately give the child positive attention. Think of your comments as sunlight that shines on positive behaviors, making them flourish. Systematic ignoring keeps negative behaviors in the dark where they can't grow.

That said, keep in mind that praising and ignoring the ADHD child in the classroom or home is not easy. The attention and comments from other students and siblings often counteract what you are trying to accomplish.

The rest of this section includes other consequences you can effectively use to augment praising and ignoring.

CALL A TIME-OUT FOR DISRUPTIVE BEHAVIOR

Even if you have used time-out previously and found it didn't work, there may be ways to increase its effectiveness. The key to time-out lies in its definition and how and when it is applied.

Remember That Time-Out Means Time-Out from Positive Reinforcement.

Your child must feel that he is losing out on something for time-out to be most effective. It may be your positive praise, your attention, or the ability to earn points in a token system. Your child should not get the impression that time-out is an opportunity to avoid a chore or responsibility.

Select Only a Few Behaviors for Which the Child Will Be Sent to Time-Out.
With the child, define in writing exactly what behaviors will result in time-out. If a child is sent to time-out for every problem behavior, it will soon lose its effectiveness.

Choose an Effective Time-Out Location.
Although time-out is a technique that may be applied wherever you are, begin by identifying a safe but boring time-out location at home and school. If you are out in public, you may elect to return to the car, where you will supervise your child for time-out.

Being sent out of the classroom may actually be reinforcing if the student gets out of work. In some households, being sent to your bedroom is as punishing as being sent to an amusement park. Under those conditions, time-out is unlikely to reduce the undesirable behavior.

Many parents find that the simplest and most effective time-out is a chair placed "away from the action." In this way the child is easily supervised and feels excluded from what else might be occurring.

Keep Time-Out Brief.
Often parents equate time-out with grounding. They send their child to time-out for extended periods such as the rest of the afternoon or evening. Time-out should be brief. The child is quickly presented with the opportunity to demonstrate the more appropriate behavior. A few minutes in a quiet corner or an isolated chair will seem like an eternity to a young, active child. A general rule of thumb is one minute of time-out for each year of age. A ten-year-old would spend ten minutes in time-out. Use a timer to signal when time-out is over, informing the youngster that if he is calmly seated when the bell rings, he may leave time-out.

Use a Clear Signal for Time-Out.
Use a "one, two, three" system to clearly indicate that time-out is imminent if the behavior continues. If you give a first warning, say, "That is one," and hold one finger up so that the youngster can see it. If a second signal is necessary, both say the number and hold up two fingers. On three, say, "That is three, time-out," as you hold up three fingers. Of course, there are times when a child should not get three chances. Some behavior, such as a sock in the arm to a sibling, may call for an automatic

"three" and an immediate time-out. In any case, when time-out is earned, the child should immediately go to the time-out location.

Maintain the Child in Time-Out.

Many times parents ask, "What do you do when a child will not stay in the time-out chair?" For each act of resistance, the child should earn another minute in time-out, but no more than a few minutes should be added to the total. A small child can be held in the time-out seat by placing your hands firmly on his shoulders. Physical restraint may antagonize some children and is not a good idea for older children in any case. In those situations, other consequences should be used, such as loss of a privilege. Being unable to enforce time-out may be an indication your child is out of control in other ways. Accept this as a sign you should seek additional professional help to learn more effective management skills.

IMMEDIATELY REPRIMAND THE CHILD FOR OFF-TASK BEHAVIOR AND DISRUPTIONS

ADHD youngsters need more positive and negative consequences than other children to change their behavior. Studies show that the correct use of reprimands can be even more effective than praising and ignoring in decreasing off-task and disruptive behavior. You may be surprised to learn that research also indicates that ADHD youth are sensitive to reprimands that pertain to their interactions with peers. Dr. Ann Abramowitz of Emory University found evidence that immediate short reprimands for interactions with other students decreased the amount of student-to-student off-task behavior. However, these teacher actions had little effect on noninteractive off-task behavior. Other studies have found that sudden, strong reprimands for disruptive behavior could also be effective in decreasing unwanted behaviors.

Make Specific Reprimands in a Firm but Calm Voice Immediately Following the Behavior.

A number of research studies have found that even a brief delay between disruptive behavior and a reprimand lessens its effectiveness. In addition, the reprimands should be given in a firm but calm voice.

Before voicing a reprimand, get the child's attention and make eye contact. With a younger child, you may want to touch the child's shoulder or even orient the child toward you. This would not be appropriate with an older youth or adolescent, and it might anger a particularly oppositional youngster.

As with praise, each reprimand should be a comment on the child's behavior, not personality. Avoid statements about the child or his character, such as, "You are bad," or even, "You are doing bad." State in very specific terms what your child is doing wrong. For example, a teacher might say, "You are out of your seat during work time. Sit down now." If your child is hitting his brother, you could remark, "Stop hitting your brother, sit back down, and work on your math homework, now!"

TRY TOKEN REINFORCEMENT IN THE CLASSROOM

In a classic study conducted in 1975, Dr. Teodoro Ayllon and colleagues at Georgia State University showed how token reinforcement given for academic work completed in the classroom can decrease disruptive behaviors as significantly as medication. Over the years, numerous additional studies have shown the effectiveness of using token systems with ADHD and other students to manage various types of learning and behavior problems.

A token reinforcement system can be used effectively at both home and school to increase on-task behaviors and to decrease disruptive behaviors. For younger children, using actual tokens such as colored chips is more effective than using symbolic points, while older children typically respond better to a more "sophisticated" point system. Dr. Michael Gordon has developed an automated reinforcement system employed in various classrooms around the United States that permits a teacher to award points by remote control. The child has an automated counter on his desk. When the teacher observes that he is on-task for the desired time she electronically adds one point to his counter.

There are several key elements involved in the creation of a successful token system.

Clearly Define the Behaviors for Which a Youngster May Earn Tokens.
Write the rules for earning tokens in positive terms. For example, "Each math page completed earns one point." Review these rules often.

**Award Tokens or Points to the Child as Soon as Possible
Following the Desired Behavior.**

For the youngster to make a connection between the desired behavior
and the positive consequences, the two events must occur in close prox-
imity. Promises that you will pay the child "later" have little meaning.

**Designate a Regular Time for the Child to Spend or Trade in Points
for Items on a Menu of Rewards.**

There should be a number of desirable rewards available at different
costs. The reward menu should include a selection of material rewards
and activities or privileges. Any system in which children have so many
points that they don't need any more or have nothing to spend them on
will break down.

Children Should Earn More Points Than They Lose.

A number of studies have indicated that in addition to awarding tokens
for positive behaviors, taking away tokens for negative behaviors can be
an effective intervention. However, if the youngster begins to lose more
tokens than he earns, the system will break down and must be modified.

Use Response Cost.

An alternative to taking away points earned is to develop a *response cost*
system. In a response cost system the child receives a specific number of
tokens at the beginning of each day or session. Tokens are then taken
away for inappropriate behaviors. This approach has been found to be
effective in suppressing disruptive behaviors.

SET UP A HOME-SCHOOL FEEDBACK SYSTEM

There are a number of advantages to using a home-school feedback system. First and foremost, the parent receives daily information about the
child's behavior in school. This provides an opportunity to reinforce
progress or solve problems if difficulties continue. Second, although a
token system is a very effective approach to improving the ADHD child's
behavior, it takes skill, time, and effort to implement effectively. Many
teachers are simply too busy to create or to conduct a school-based token
system for one or two students. With daily feedback, it is up to the parent
to provide effective reinforcement or consequences. Since the parent

maintains control of many of the most effective reinforcers—such as television, video games, time with friends, and time with parents—a home-school feedback system provides an effective way to administer them.

There are several points to keep in mind when you create a home-school feedback system:

Keep It Simple.

Two reporting forms are shown below. Figure 4.1 shows a Daily Report appropriate for a younger child. The data are easy for the teacher to provide, since information about only two behaviors is collected in a very simple way. Did the child sit in his seat as was appropriate for none, some, most, or all of the day? Did the child complete none, some, most, or almost all of his work? A Summary Report form like the one in Figure 4.2 is appropriate for an older child or adolescent and could be sent home daily or weekly. It provides information about the same two behaviors but in a more sophisticated manner. The behaviors could be adapted for individual children depending on what type of behavior you are attempting to build.

Make It Easy for the Teacher.

You may copy the forms provided in Figure 4.1 and 4.2 to set up a home-school feedback system. Regardless of the form you use, make and date enough copies for the teacher to send home for several weeks. When you are first introducing the system to your child, reward him for simply bringing home a report each day, in addition to whatever points he earns for behavior.

Clarify the Behaviors That Are Being Tracked.

Before initiating the system, have a meeting with the teacher and your child to discuss specific goals and how the system is to be carried out. For students who have more than one teacher, you may have one teacher orchestrate the system or have all the teachers present.

It is important that each person's responsibilities be clearly defined. For younger children, the teacher will be responsible for remembering to fill out the form and send it home. However, your child will still be responsible for bringing home the card or record. Older children should assume greater responsibility. They may be required to supply the form to the teacher. Sometimes the student is asked to record his own behavior; then the teacher simply verifies the information with his signature or initials.

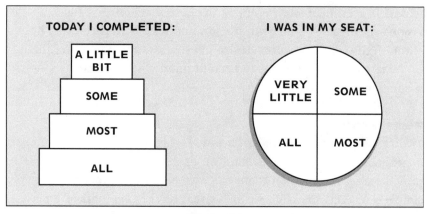

Figure 4.1
Daily Report

Promptly Reinforce Earned Behaviors.
It is very effective when the home-school feedback report serves as the child's "ticket" to an evening's event or activities. For example, for having completed at least most of his work that day, the student might be allowed to watch television or play a video game. In essence, the consequences become automatic: No report, no television. Or if the child did not successfully fulfill his part of the agreement, he does not earn the designated privileges.

THE ADHD ADULT AT WORK

If you are an adult who has been struggling with ADHD all your life, you are likely to intuitively know much about the kind of environments in which you function best. You have probably learned a lot of this the hard way: by trial and error. Weiss and Hechtman of Montreal Children's Hospital, in their retroactive studies of ADHD adults grown up, found that these adults had changed jobs more often than their non-ADHD counterparts. Many ADHD adults fail because the same behaviors that plagued them in regimented school settings follow them to the workplace.

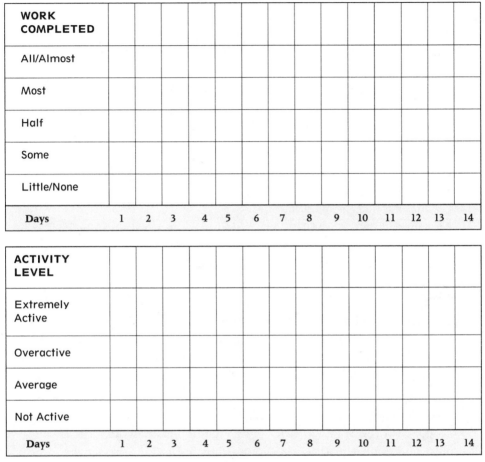

WORK COMPLETED														
All/Almost														
Most														
Half														
Some														
Little/None														
Days	1	2	3	4	5	6	7	8	9	10	11	12	13	14

ACTIVITY LEVEL														
Extremely Active														
Overactive														
Average														
Not Active														
Days	1	2	3	4	5	6	7	8	9	10	11	12	13	14

Figure 4.2
Summary Report

EVALUATE YOUR WORK STYLE AND KNOW YOUR WEAKNESSES

Most often, successful ADHD adults have found positions that fit their style or have made changes to the work environment that compensate for their weaknesses. George was a natural-born salesman. But his distractibility, impulsiveness, and disorganization worked against him. Often on beautiful afternoons he'd decide on the spur of the moment to play a game of tennis rather than seek out new clients. The gift of gab worked for and against him. He could sell anything to anyone, but sometimes he'd get distracted and forget to present a new product. That cost him money. Finally, he got a terrific secretary. She made his appointments and kept him on schedule. He told her how many calls a day he wanted to make, and she kept a running count. She also made sure he had in hand the materials about each new product before making a call.

You may know a good deal about your work style. As you think about your work situation, consider whether you have set up the optimum situation for the various elements of your job over which you have control.

CHANGE YOUR PHYSICAL ENVIRONMENT AT THE OFFICE

Consider the Placement of Your Desk.

For some adults with ADHD, where their desk is at work can be just as important as where a student sits in class. Draw a mental picture of your work space, including windows, doors, and other desks. Now consider the types of spaces where you are the most productive. Where do you go when you want to read a great book or have written work that you must get done? In school, where did you study best: in the carrels in the back of the library, or an isolated room? When you need to complete a task that requires concentration, where do you go?

Jerome has learned how he works best. A stockbroker by day, he functions well in the hustle-bustle environment of his brokerage firm as long as making phone calls to collect information and to contact clients is his goal. However, he has determined that to dictate, write, or read, he must find a quiet place where he can turn his back to the activity and noise.

What about your desk? Do you face the door and continue to keep your door open to everyone who walks by? That may be great for developing camaraderie in the office, but is it good for the work effort? Some ADHD adults find that positioning the desk away from the door and toward a wall is imperative if they are going to get anything done.

An executive we worked with resisted turning his back to the door, but once he did, it worked so well he got a promotion. Unfortunately, the perk that came with the promotion was a new, corner office with a wonderful view of the park. He enjoyed people-watching, but his work suffered until he turned his desk around. Even then he was tempted to sneak more than a few peaks, especially in the spring.

Consider the Size and Clutter of Your Work Space.

Think about the room in which you work. Some adults simply cannot function in a large open space. Even a glass cubicle offers very little shield. Being able to hear the sounds around them and to see their co-workers is simply too distracting. For these people, having an office with a door that can be shut is not a status symbol or a luxury, but a necessity.

It is important to recognize how stacked papers, incomplete work, books, pencils, telephones, faxes, and the other tools and products of today's work environment impinge upon your ability to get something done. Like the student who is overwhelmed by too many papers in his work folder, the image of a staggering workload staring you in the face may slow your progress. You may simply function better in a clean work space or a bare room.

Eliminating the visual and auditory distractions is not everyone's answer to productivity. It may help some ADHD sufferers, but others need a lot of stimulation to stay alert. If you fall into this category, you may thrive on the hustle and bustle of a large, busy work space like a newsroom or TV station. You may prefer the kind of job where the setting is constantly changing as you move from appointment to appointment. You may work best under ever-changing deadlines or news flashes. For example, some stockbrokers flourish in the fluid environment of the ticker tape flashing, the phone ringing, and clients going and coming. Sitting in a quiet office with no stimulation would actually lead to a decrease in efficiency and work output. A young ADHD disk jockey–talk show host we met in Boston said it best, "I have to have the lights, noise, and constant stimulation of the control room—instant choices and changes, music going, commercials to run, telephones ringing, and lights blinking. I thrive on it."

Work Near Coworkers Who Make Your Efforts Better.

As in school, your neighbor can be a bonus or a detriment to the work effort. You will find that there are coworkers whose work style is a boon to yours. For example, you may be the creative thinker in the crowd, so pairing yourself with a linear thinker who is very organized may enhance both of your efforts.

There are two people in the office who can have a major influence on your success. The first is your supervisor; the second is your assistant. One salesman we worked with was quite productive as long as he had a boss who supervised him closely and a secretary who followed through on his efforts. Unfortunately, when this young man took a new position, the new company had a different work philosophy and with much less of a team approach. Each salesman kept his own records and followed up on his own sales. Without supervision and follow-through, the young man's productivity and income took an immediate plunge. Luckily, he quickly realized his mistake and was able to return to his old job, where he went on to become a sales manager. With his same secretary next door and his old boss, who was now a vice president and still a mentor, he remained a successful employee.

CHANGE YOUR WORK SCHEDULE

As when you were a student, planning your work schedule to fit your style is very important. Janet is a thirty-two-year-old lawyer who had trouble reading briefs, contracts, and other lengthy documents. At first, she scheduled her mornings for meetings, clients, and conference calls, her afternoons for reading and writing. This led to problems, so she scheduled her mornings in the firm's law library and used the afternoons for meetings. She found that this change led to major improvements in her efficiency.

If your job allows you to alter your schedule, play with the types of activities you assign to various parts of the day. Just because you have "always" done something one way doesn't mean it is the best way.

THE ADHD ADULT WORKING AT HOME

Few adults find working at home easy. Unless you've planned for a home business and taught your family what that means, it's tough to work at home. However, when ADHD adults bring work home that they were unable to complete in the office, it takes extra effort and finesse to get the work accomplished.

IDENTIFY AN ADULT WORK SPACE

Whether it's a table in the kitchen, a desk in the bedroom, or a full-fledged home office, you need a clearly defined place to work at home. This will help you keep up with ongoing tasks, such as paying bills or completing work that is brought home from the office. Most ADHD adults find it is essential to have a cleared, isolated spot in the house to do such work. A few, though, discover that the seclusion sends their minds wandering. In the latter case, you're better off sitting at a cleared table in the kitchen or den than at a desk in the study or bedroom.

SET ASIDE TIME TO WORK

Even when you are not ADHD, finding the time to work is a problem. There's always someone or something competing for attention. That problem is compounded several times over when you are ADHD. It is imperative to schedule time to pay bills, make phone calls, or meet other deadlines. Use a sign to notify everyone in the house—including your-self—that this is the time allotted to a particular task and that you are not to be disturbed.

CHANGE THE TASK TO INCREASE PRODUCTIVITY

We know that people with ADHD can become easily overwhelmed by the work they must do. We know that students, for example, work more productively when their assignments are presented in smaller, more manageable workloads. At least for the student, teachers and parents can serve as "traffic cops" to control the flow of work. In the real world of work, where events, deadlines, and crises are often unforeseen and be-yond our control, restructuring our daily work is not quite as easy. Many of the same principles of work organization still apply, though, and even though you are grown up, you might want to browse through the previ-ous section of this chapter for some helpful hints.

While you probably cannot determine how and when assignments come to you, you can become familiar with your own strengths and weaknesses and try to reorganize your workday to your best advantage.

Take on Only One Assignment at a Time.

The allotment of tasks, as outlined earlier for students, can be an effective technique at work too. You may discover that when your supervisor gives you one task with a clear estimate of how long it should take, you are able to work much more efficiently. Similarly, even if you are a boss who has trouble prioritizing, a very organized secretary or assistant can dole out incoming items a few at a time.

Break the Workload into Smaller Parts.

Earlier, on page 66, we explained how to divide assignments into smaller parts for students. This strategy can sometimes work for ADHD adults. Many adult sufferers become overwhelmed by the simplest projects. To overcome this, break each task down into doable components. *Doable* in this case means whatever is manageable at the time. For example, one mother of the bride was finding it difficult to deal with the endless list of details for her daughter's wedding. (As any mother of the bride can tell you, you don't need to have ADHD to be overwhelmed by that!) Her first step was to work with a friend who had planned her own daughter's wedding, making a checklist of all the jobs she would need to do as well as an estimation of when to do each. Certain tasks, however, particularly frightened her—for example, addressing three hundred wedding invitations. The task became much less intimidating and easier to handle when she decided to address the invitations one letter of the alphabet at a time. In between sessions of doing that, she worked on smaller, less overwhelming tasks.

Alter or Reduce the Written Workload.

We've long known that any task that involves writing can be difficult for a student with ADHD; we've seen in recent years how well many of them respond to working with a computer. If writing is still a challenge for you, you might consider dictating reports and correspondence. Using a word processing program on a computer not only makes dealing with the written word generally easier but also eliminates problems with handwriting and spelling.

IMPROVE ATTENTION TO DETAILS

Attention to details is likely to have been a bugaboo for you all your life. Your spouse and friends may tease you about your inattention, and coworkers may simply have labeled you a ''big picture'' guy. You can train yourself to note details. Some of the same suggestions made on page 67 for students will work as you read reports and other documents. Ask family members, friends, and coworkers to make sure they have your attention before giving you information or making a request. Get in the habit of repeating directions told to you. Adopt a scanning technique we call the "hesitation response" (see page 171) to improve your memory for details. When you enter or leave a room, scan the environment and yourself, noting items you will need or have left behind.

A FINAL WORD ON WHAT TO TRY BEFORE YOU TRY MEDICATION

As you can see, there are many things you can try before you decide to place your child or yourself on medication. For some individuals with mild symptoms, or those whose problems are identified very early, this may be all the intervention needed for a while or forever. For others, applying every intervention we've discussed in an effective, consistent manner will not bring about the desired results. For those individuals, it is certainly appropriate—even desirable—to try medication. We cannot overemphasize what research and past experience bear out: *A combined approach of behavioral intervention and medication is more effective in reducing disruptive behavior, increasing attention, and modifying many of the problems associated with ADHD than either medication or behavioral approaches alone.*

In our first book on ADHD, *If Your Child Is Hyperactive, Inattentive, Impulsive, Distractible . . . ,* we presented a training program based on our work with hundreds of children at our clinic. These approaches along with those of other professionals may provide the assistance your child needs to manage the day-to-day problems of ADHD. Use the checklist that follows to guide your efforts to bring about behavioral change before trying medication.

THINGS TO TRY BEFORE YOU TRY MEDICATION

RESTRUCTURE THE ENVIRONMENT
____ 1. Change where child sits in the classroom (front, back, isolated).
____ 2. If possible, change the type of classroom (structured/specialized).
____ 3. If possible, change schools (smaller/specialized).

PROVIDE GOOD MODELS
____ 1. Place the student next to appropriate role model(s).
____ 2. Pair the student with a "study buddy" to verify directions and assignments.
____ 3. Do projects with organized partner(s).

ALTER THE TIME OF WORK
____ 1. Arrange the class schedule to reflect student's best time of day.
____ 2. Change homework/study time.

RESTRUCTURE TASKS
____ 1. Assign one task at a time.
____ 2. Break assignments into smaller parts.
____ 3. Circle key words in instructions.
____ 4. Have student make eye contact and repeat oral directions.
____ 5. Reduce the amount of copying and written work required.
____ 6. Allow student to use alternative modes to show knowledge.
____ 7. Use the computer whenever possible for written expression, drill, and practice.

IMPLEMENT BEHAVIORAL INTERVENTIONS
____ 1. Use systematic praise and ignoring.
____ 2. Give immediate reprimands for off-task behaviors.
____ 3. Use token reinforcement.
____ 4. Set up a home-school feedback-reinforcement system.
____ 5. Use time-outs for disruptive behaviors.

5

WHEN MEDICATION IS NEEDED

Finding the Best Fit

Before deciding to use medication for ADHD, you and your physician, psychologist, or psychiatrist should be sure you have taken all the steps to get an accurate diagnosis of ADHD (see Chapter 3). Once that's been confirmed and you or your child has tried alternative approaches to the problem unsuccessfully, you face an important decision. Whether an adult determining a course of action for yourself or the parent of a child whose future rests in your hands, your deciding to try medication is a major step. In view of how little we professionals can offer in terms of accurate prognosis and reassurances about outcomes, we must respect the courage and tenacity of people with ADHD and parents of ADHD youngsters. Whether they end up taking medication for a short time or for the rest of their lives; whether they experience dramatic, positive results or see only incremental improvements; whether we somehow hit on the perfect regimen immediately or it eludes us through periods of trial and error, beginning medication is fraught with potential satisfaction and disappointment, breakthroughs and frustration. Every new prescription for ADHD medication is like an incomplete map: Only the person taking the medication can tell us where it will take him, and then only after he has arrived.

That said, it's important to bear in mind that for many people who do try medication, the decision proves to be the right one. Since there's no way to determine that beforehand, it's especially important that you approach this "journey," as it were, from the right perspective. Be prepared:

- Work only with professionals you trust and who have had extensive experience treating people with ADHD.

- Educate yourself about the possible risks and side effects of every medication used for ADHD. Understand that different medications are often prescribed in combination, to treat specific symptoms.
- Discuss with the prescribing professional issues of concern, such as past problems with drug abuse (which do not automatically rule out medication to treat ADHD), or a family history of Tourette's syndrome or tics.

Living with ADHD is never easy. Coping with it, with or without medication, requires commitment and the willingness to try new things. Using medication is no different. The decision to try medication may come at the end of a long road, but it is not a destination in itself, only another beginning.

MAKING CHOICES ABOUT MEDICATION

CHUCK's parents had tried everything before considering medication. When they agreed with their son's teacher, psychologist, and pediatrician that it was time to try medication, they thought Ritalin was the only choice. After increasing the dosage, and finding that Ritalin still didn't yield a positive response, they were very discouraged. However, Chuck was switched to Dexedrine and there was an immediate, noticeable change in behavior, with fewer side effects.

Ritalin is not the only drug prescribed for ADHD, just the best known. Whether prescribed by the brand name Ritalin or in its generic form, methylphenidate, it is taken by more ADHD children and adults than any other medication. That computes to about 70 percent of the school-age children diagnosed with ADHD in this country. Other children and adults diagnosed with ADHD may take Ritalin SR, Dexedrine, Cylert, or a number of other medications for their particular set of problems.

There are choices that must be made in order to find the best fit of medication for yourself or your child. Of course, your physician must prescribe medication. The treatment team—the physician, your child, the teacher, and the psychologist or other professionals for the child; or your physician, psychologist, spouse, or friends—will provide guidance, but they will depend on feedback from you. In selecting a medication, the following points should be kept in mind.

INDIVIDUAL RESPONSES TO MEDICATION VARY

A child's or an adult's response to medication is highly variable and unpredictable. Attempts to predict who will respond positively to medication based on overt aspects of behavior have not been successful. Several researchers report the shorter an individual's attention span, the more likely she will respond to medication. Dr. Russell Barkley has also reported, on the basis of his research, that the greater the child-mother bond, the more likely the child will respond to medication.

A factor that appears to be related to a child's response to medication is whether the ADHD individual is hyperactive. Some studies indicate a greater percentage of children who are ADHD without hyperactivity do not respond to methylphenidate.

We are only beginning to understand how the brain processes information and which parts of the information-processing chain may be interrupted or impaired in ADHD. In recent years, researchers' understanding of the neurochemistry of the brain has grown greatly, but many individuals diagnosed as ADHD vary greatly in the characteristics they exhibit. Your child may be extremely overactive; another child may be highly impulsive and inattentive but not overly active. It is possible that each aspect of ADHD reflects a different aspect of brain function and a distinct level of neurochemical mediation. If this is true, then it is also likely that an individual's response to medication varies because of the distinct areas of the brain and equally different aspects of neurochemical activity affected by medication.

In general, most people studying ADHD agree that about 25 percent of children or adults who try stimulants report no effects. That doesn't mean there's anything wrong with the child or adult, or that the bond between parent and child is not strong enough. *It simply means that stimulants did not work for that individual.*

BE METHODICAL; TAKE AMPLE TIME TO FIND
THE RIGHT DOSE AND MEDICATION

The first medication you try may not work, but it is even more likely that the first dosage tried will not be the right one. There is no single dosage that will be appropriate for everyone. Your physician will set a schedule of trial dosages for you or your child. It is important to follow the schedule exactly and to gather information about you or your child's response to each level of medication.

Your child will be able to give you a lot of information about his response to medication—through either words or actions. An older child is especially able to tell you about differences in how he feels or is able to function on medication. Kyle at first reported that he noticed little difference as he began a trial of Ritalin. His first recognized response was that he bettered his best time on a one-mile run at school because he was not daydreaming, but was concentrating on his goal. With later doses and increases in medication, he was able to accurately observe improved note-taking in class, better attention, and less distractibility. His reaction—"This is the right dose for me!"—was a key in determining the optimum medication dosage.

When your child is at home, you can be the observer, but when your child is at school, you need the teacher's help. Getting consistent feedback about a child's performance in the classroom is invaluable in determining the appropriate medication.

When you do find the best fit for medication, everyone will know it. Teachers will report improvement in certain areas of behavior, the child or adult will feel more in control, and you will note positive responses. You can then weigh the side effects and make appropriate decisions with the aid of your physician.

UNDERSTANDING THE MEDICATIONS FOR ADHD

You will never need most of the medications we will discuss. However, it is important for you to know what the alternatives are and how they differ. Our goal here is not to make you a pharmacologist or a physician. We want to provide enough information so that you can ask the right questions and make better choices for your child or yourself.

Of course, the reasons you would try medication are the positive effects associated with attention, academic performance, and other areas of behavior. These will be discussed in detail in the appropriate chapters of this book.

STIMULANTS

The psychostimulants associated with ADHD are Ritalin (methylphenidate); Dexedrine (dextroamphetamine), and Cylert (pemoline).

In general, most physicians recommend that Ritalin or its generic equivalent, methylphenidate, be tried first. Many people believe that methylphenidate is slightly less effective than Ritalin. However, there is no conclusive evidence to support the belief.

Josephine Elia and Judith Rapoport, from the National Institutes of Mental Health, suggest that both Ritalin and Dexedrine (dextroamphetamine) should be given on a trial basis before choosing one over the other. Both drugs have been proven effective in treating ADHD, although some prefer dextroamphetamine, probably because it has a longer response time.

Each of these medications is taken orally and is quickly absorbed through the gastrointestinal tract into the bloodstream. Both Ritalin and Dexedrine come in fast-acting and time-release forms.

How They Work

It is generally accepted that stimulant medications increase the alertness or arousal of the central nervous system. Exactly how they do this is still not totally understood, but quite consistently now the literature is defining ADHD as a disorder of the neurotransmitters in the brain.

The brain is made of millions and millions of neurons across which stimuli or electrical messages travel. Put very simply, stimuli must travel from one neuron to another across a tiny gap called the *synapse*. Once it reaches the synapse, the electrical signal causes the release of a chemical called a *neurotransmitter* from the ends of the neuron, the *axon*. Once the neurotransmitter is released and absorbed by the proper receptors on the other side of the synapse, the signal can bridge the gap. Without the neurotransmitters, the relay of stimuli is impossible.

The movement of impulses across the synapses is the physiological mechanism by which our brains "learn." Every activity requires the movement of electrical impulses across a neuron path. For example, when you learn to play a piano piece, electrical impulses must make their way from the fingers to the brain and back again. With each practice session, the trip by the electrical impulses along the pathway becomes better established and the piano piece can be played more fluently. Learning occurs after an electrical impulse produced by a stimulus is transmitted and moves across a neuron-synaptic course several times. (This explains why repetition is so important.) With practice or repetition, the path is believed to become automatic. Once established, these automatic pathways last forever. If in ADHD these neural bridges are blocked or incomplete, whatever is being learned does not become automatic.

To complicate the story, there are many different neurotransmitters. Each one matches up to a different receptor on the other side of the synapse. Researchers have discovered that various deficiencies in different transmitters create distinct problems. For example, Parkinson's disease results from a deficiency in dopamine; acetylcholine seems to play a role in Alzheimer's; and Tourette's syndrome may indicate a problem with dopamine also. The neurotransmitters that are most often cited as playing a role in ADHD are *norepinephrine* and *dopamine.*

Some of the medications that are used to treat ADHD, such as Ritalin and Dexedrine, increase the availability of neurotransmitters before the synapse; other medications, such as some antidepressants, work to prevent the reuptake, or reabsorption, of the neurotransmitter after its release. For example, most researchers are clearest about how dextroamphetamine, better known as d-amphetamine, works in the brain. D-amphetamine helps by increasing the availability of two neurotransmitters, norepinephrine and/or dopamine, at the synapse between neurons in certain areas of the brain.

Side Effects of Stimulant Medication

Every medication has side effects. You may not experience them, or you may have an initial reaction that goes away within a few days. Sometimes, however, a severe or unexpected reaction occurs. Should this happen to you or your child, discuss the matter immediately with your physician. Medication should always be monitored on a regular basis through observation and reports from the ADHD individual, teachers, parents, and others. You will want to collect information about appetite, sleep patterns, repetitive or ticlike motions, and other problematic characteristics of ADHD and remain abreast of new research on the use of medication for ADHD. We will discuss the monitoring process later in this chapter. Some medications like Cylert will require regular blood tests to monitor side effects.

The most common and best-known side effects of stimulant medications are loss of appetite and insomnia. Other negative side effects, such as headaches, stomachaches, and on rare occasions constipation, fluctuate with the dosage and typically either are not severe enough to warrant stopping treatment or go away after a period of time.

Ritalin has been studied worldwide for more than thirty years. At the present time, there is no conclusive evidence of long-term negative life-threatening side effects in individuals taking Ritalin and other stimulants over long periods of time. In 1991, Dr. Robert Diener, senior advisor, Licensing and Safety Evaluation, Ciba-Geigy, completely reviewed the toxicology studies of Ritalin and confidently commented on the rare number of recorded adverse reactions to this medication. Even reports of adverse reaction to purposeful overdosages of methylphenidate or intravenous exposure to this drug are rare.

It is interesting to note that in the research studies, irritability, anxiety, and crying, which are commonly associated with medication, are also reported when individuals are taking a placebo. Since oversensitivity is a characteristic symptom of ADHD itself, it is difficult to attribute it to drug treatment alone.

There are several drug-related side effects that you should be aware of and should carefully monitor. A very small group of children treated with stimulant medication, perhaps 1 percent, may display repetitive movements, or tics, such as blinking, finger playing, or shoulder shrugging. If there is a personal history of Tourette's syndrome or if it runs in your family, the tics may increase with medication. If you notice such actions or have a history of Tourette's syndrome, you should discuss the matter immediately with your doctor. Most often, any tics that occur as a result of medication will fade after the drug treatment is discontinued.

The most discussed side effect of stimulant medication is height and weight suppression. Appetite loss appears to be more of a problem with dextroamphetamine than methylphenidate and occurs more noticeably at higher doses. Numerous studies have shown that stimulants probably do not have long-term, permanent effects. A growth rebound typically occurs after the first year of treatment and during drug-free holiday periods. Studies of ADHD adults who took medication as children have not confirmed long-term decreases in height or weight. One study, conducted by Drs. Mattes and Gittelman and reported in the *Archives of General Psychiatry* in 1983, found a slight decrease in height after an individual took methylphenidate for a number of years. The researchers emphasized that the decrease in height was related to the total amount of medication taken during a yearly period. This problem appears to be eliminated if the drug is discontinued for catch-up periods, during which growth may occur.

Rebound Effects

A final side effect that is important to note is the "rebound effect." The rebound effect denotes a period of time—usually in the late afternoon, although it also may occur between 11:30 A.M. and 12 noon—during which a child is irritable and reactive. Although many people assume this befalls all children on medication, actually only 30 percent of the children who take stimulants experience it.

Most often studied in relation to methylphenidate, the rebound effect seems to vary across individuals and across days. One child may never experience a rebound effect; another may have rebound effects several afternoons of the week and not others. Usually a smaller dose of methylphenidate at noon or a small dose of the medication in the late afternoon will reduce the severity of the rebound without affecting evening appetite or sleep. If you observe this pattern in your child, discuss the proper course of action with your physician.

Ritalin

Ritalin gets all the blame and most of the accolades when it comes to medications for ADHD. When it works well, it has been called a wonder drug. However, as you are discovering, there are no miracles when it comes to ADHD. No drug cures ADHD.

The effects of Ritalin are usually noted within thirty to sixty minutes after taking the medication. Peak effects occur within one to three hours, and most influences are gone within three to five hours. The drug is entirely metabolized and out of the body within twelve to twenty-four hours.

Typically Ritalin is first given in a 5 mg dosage at breakfast and, perhaps, at noon. The initial dose may be 10 mg for older, larger children, adolescents, or adults. Dosages are increased by steps of 2.5 or 5 mg until the appropriate dose is established. Once the optimum dose is found, it is usually administered twice a day.

The sustained-release form of Ritalin, Ritalin SR, has effects that last from four to six hours and sometimes as much as seven or eight hours. The influences of the medication are usually noted within one to two hours of ingestion, with optimum performance occurring within three to five hours. Most effects have vanished within eight hours after taking the medication.

The sustained-release form of methylphenidate, Ritalin SR, shows greater variability across individuals. In addition, many people report that the effects of Ritalin SR also vary with what the individual eats during the day. That is why many physicians prefer to dispense Ritalin in its short-acting form. If a sustained-release medication is desired, most people turn to Dexedrine.

Dexedrine

Dexedrine also comes in short-acting and sustained-release forms. The short-acting form is commonly used to find the appropriate dose of medication. Once that is established, the time-release form is often substituted.

The behavioral effects of Dexedrine are typically noted within thirty to sixty minutes after consumption, and peak within one to two hours. Most effects are gone within four to six hours. However, it is not unusual for individuals to vary in their response to Dexedrine.

Direct comparisons of Dexedrine and Ritalin in the literature are few. As mentioned earlier, Drs. Elia and Rapoport strongly believe both medications should be tried before one or the other is chosen. Studies that have compared the medications have found both drugs to reduce motor restlessness, but individual responses to one medication or the other may differ.

Generally speaking, milligram for milligram, Dexedrine is considered to be twice as strong as Ritalin. Therefore, if a child was taking Ritalin previously, a physician might begin a trial dose of Dexedrine at half the dose of Ritalin. Again, Dexedrine would be prescribed in steps of 2.5 mg until the optimum dosage is established.

Eight-year-old Toby had taken Ritalin for a number of months with no noticeable improvement in behavior. When it was decided to try Dexedrine, Toby's doctor began with an initial dosage half of his last dose of Ritalin. Since Toby had last taken 10 mg of Ritalin twice a day, he was now advised to take 5 mg of the short-acting form of Dexedrine after breakfast and at 12:00 noon.

Toby's parents were given the following schedule to guide their administration of medication: They were told to write down any effects they or Toby noticed on a page like the one shown in Figure 5.1. If any effects, positive or negative, were noted, they were discussed with the doctor before continuing.

Cylert

Cylert, whose main ingredient is pemoline, is similar in treatment effects to Ritalin or Dexedrine, but it has a longer period of effectiveness during the day. Unlike Ritalin and Dexedrine, Cylert takes a number of weeks

MEDICATION: DEXEDRINE, SHORT-ACTING			
DAY	7 A.M.	12:00 P.M.	COMMENTS
1	5 mg		
2	5 mg		
3	7.5 mg		
4	7.5 mg		
5	10 mg	5 mg	
6	10 mg	5 mg	

Figure 5.1
Comments on Medication

for its maximum effects to be seen. This slow building-up effect makes adjustments in dosage for Cylert more difficult. However, the longer-acting characteristic can lead to more stable functioning without rebound effects. Also, since the medication is taken only once a day, compliance issues can be minimized.

Cylert is available in capsules of 18.75, 37.5, and 75 mg. Dosage varies between 0.5 and 3 mg/kg. It is typically administered once a day with initial doses starting at 18.75 mg, with a dosage range of 37.5 to 112.5 mg/day. Once the optimum dose is found, it is usually taken once a day.

You should be aware that beyond the side effects typically associated with other stimulant medications discussed previously, Cylert has been shown to occasionally adversely affect liver function. For this reason, it is important to monitor liver function in anyone taking Cylert.

ANTIDEPRESSANTS

Tricyclic antidepressants are slower-acting medications that have been shown to be effective in decreasing inattention, hyperactivity, and aggression for some children. Although less extensively researched than the stimulants, antidepressants such as imipramine (Tofranil) and desipramine (Norpramin) do not appear to have any influence—either positive or negative—on cognitive functioning. Since the effect appears to be more pinpointed to specific neurotransmitters, they may have some advantage in treating very hyperactive youth. In addition, the antidepressants offer a longer period of effectiveness without a rebound effect, greater flexibility in dosage, and minimal risk of drug abuse.

In general, the antidepressants remain a secondary choice of medication for those with ADHD. However, if a child does not show a response to the central nervous system (CNS) stimulants, antidepressants have been helpful to approximately 70 percent of these children who are nonresponders. The same may be true for adults.

There is one time when antidepressants may be a better first choice of medication. When a child or adult experiences enuresis, or bed-wetting, has problems with moods, is highly anxious or depressed, and has a diagnosis of ADHD, he or she may show greater response to the antidepressants than to stimulant medication, or to stimulant medication used in combination with antidepressants.

Side Effects of Antidepressants

Antidepressant side effects may include dry mouth, increases in blood pressure and heart rate, and slowing of intracardiac conduction. Although these side effects are not usually a problem, anyone taking these medications should have cardiac function monitored regularly.

Imipramine

Imipramine has been used since the mid-1970s for ADHD. Some studies have shown that imipramine can decrease hyperactivity and defiance and increase sociability. Unfortunately, it often has greater side effects than methylphenidate, including increased or decreased appetite, fatigue, and increased blood pressure. Anyone taking imipramine must be closely monitored for blood pressure and cardiac side effects. A baseline EKG should be obtained before beginning a child on this medication.

Desipramine

A number of studies have shown desipramine to improve the behavior of ADHD boys. However there are reports of cardiovascular side effects, which were statistically significant but still extremely rare, including increased blood pressure, heart rate, and EKG conduction. Five deaths associated with desipramine have been reported in the literature, and many physicians now avoid using it.

There may be times when desipramine may be a very positive choice of medication for children with tics and ADHD. Several studies show that this medication is safe and effective for ADHD associated with a tic disorder, since it does not exacerbate the tics. However, any child or adult using this medication should be monitored for the side effects mentioned above.

Nortriptyline

Not widely used for ADHD, nortriptyline appears to prevent the reuptake of the neurotransmitters serotonin and acetylcholine. It has been shown to have a positive impact on attitude, attention span, and impulsivity in ADHD adolescents who had not responded to stimulants.

Other Antidepressants

A number of other antidepressants have been used with ADHD youngsters or adults. Bupropion, or Wellbutrin, and Prozac have been reportedly used either alone or in combination to improve various aspects of ADHD. Studies are beginning to indicate that these medications may positively affect ADHD characteristics. It is believed that these antidepressants may be helpful in treating ADHD youth who are highly anxious and/or depressed.

OTHER MEDICATIONS

There are a number of other medications that, although typically prescribed for other reasons, may at times be prescribed for ADHD. These medications may be used alone or in combination with a stimulant medication either to counter a particular side effect or to combat a specific problem a child or adult is having.

Clonidine

Recently, a medication used to regulate blood pressure—clonidine, or Catapres—has been effective in treating children with ADHD. Clonidine appears to have positive effects on ADHD children who are especially hyperactive, impulsive, and aggressive, and there is some indication it may be an effective choice for ADHD children with tics. It does not appear to be an effective choice for ADHD children who are predominantly ADHD inattentive type.

A positive characteristic of clonidine is that it may be administered orally or through a transdermal patch, which maintains an effective blood level of the medication for five to seven days. In addition, clonidine may improve appetite and sleep pattern. A negative side effect of clonidine is the sleepiness that occurs within an hour of administration. This side effect seems to decrease as tolerance of the medication builds over time.

Neuroleptics

Sometimes neuroleptic medications, such as haloperidol and thioridazine, have been used as adjuncts to other stimulant treatment for ADHD. While there is some empirical evidence of improvement in behavior on these medications, it is not understood why these medications may improve aspects of ADHD. More important, the side effects of involuntary movements (tardive dyskinesia) and drowsiness make the use of neuroleptics for ADHD questionable.

There are a number of additional medications that are prescribed to combat other problems that may occur along with ADHD. Please talk candidly with your physician about the potential benefits and problems associated with combining medications.

ASSESSING AND MONITORING MEDICATION

THE IMPORTANCE OF MONITORING MEDICATION

A good monitoring system helps you and the rest of the treatment team gather objective information about the effects of medication. In addition, ongoing monitoring of medication provides feedback on all areas of treatment—medical and other—so that decisions to improve it can be made. Finally, ongoing monitoring is essential to ensure the child's or adult's continued healthy and positive response to medication.

Unfortunately, often there is ineffective monitoring of medication. A survey of pediatricians conducted by Dr. Linda Copeland and her colleagues found that only 60 percent of these physicians used rating scales to assess the effects of medication. Even more disturbing was the finding that nearly 75 percent of the pediatricians relied on parents' reports *alone* to assess the effects of medications.

While parents are an important source of information about a child's response to medication, they are often not the best. Since medication is typically given in the morning and at noon, it has worn off by the time most students return home. Many families do not administer medication after school or on weekends. Without direct observation of the child's response in other settings (namely, school), you cannot provide the firsthand information needed to make decisions about medication.

As a parent, you must feel comfortable about the decision to place your child on medication. Ongoing monitoring of your child's behavior and reaction to medication will help you feel in control of the situation.

A 1982 study by Kenneth Gadow of the State University of New York examined parents' feelings about medication. Gadow found that a large number of parents did not believe their physicians spent enough time discussing the use of medication. And while communication between parents and teachers was quite frequent, crucial communication between the teacher and the physician who prescribed medication was very rare.

BEFORE BEGINNING MEDICATION

Before proceeding, we believe it important to discuss where the child fits in this decision. One of the most significant findings of the retroactive studies of ADHD adults grown up, conducted by Weiss and Hechtman at Montreal Children's Hospital during the 1970s, was the fact that ADHD adults wished someone had explained to them why they were taking medication when they were children.

In every aspect of treatment, your child or adolescent is the most important part of the treatment team. If he or she doesn't "buy into" the plan, there's a greater chance of frustration, resistance, and failure. Children need to understand ADHD, its effects, and its treatment. When you are talking to your child about ADHD, the following guidelines will be helpful:

Make Your Explanation Positive and Appropriate to the Age of the Child.

Talk to your child at his level of understanding. Avoid labels and diagnostic names. Emphasize the positive side of the symptoms. "Your mind is working so hard, it notices everything. We need to work on concentrating on what you need to attend to at the time," *not* "You just don't pay attention to what you need to." Use the concept of individual differences: "Just the way some students are better with one subject than another, some students also have a longer attention span for a particular kind of learning."

Basically, make the explanation one that helps your child relate to the symptoms. For younger elementary-age youngsters, we often use the image of "a tiger in your tank" to explain the rambunctiousness and need to move. A child who loves buses and trains might relate to the image of a runaway train.

Older youth want more information. By fourth grade, many ADHD youngsters are experiencing serious difficulty. Although diagnostic labels rarely add information to the discussion, helping youngsters to understand how individual differences play a role in their ability to work in school is crucial. When it's true, you may extend the concept to explain that you have some of the same characteristics. Using examples your child can understand, you might contrast how one parent is able to read a book in the middle of an airport, while the other has difficulty concentrating in a library. It's not anyone's fault; it just happens to be the way it is. Understanding one's weaknesses and strengths is an important step in learning how to concentrate better. A number of books that will help explain ADHD to children of various ages are listed in the Resources section.

Validate Your Child's Understanding of ADHD.

Don't underestimate your child. Children may have more information than you think they do. Make sure it is valid. You may be surprised to discover how much your child knows when you pose a few questions.

Mrs. Rosen, the mother of a boy we worked with, was quite surprised to learn just how aware her son Kenny was of his attentional problems. He certainly recognized the problem on the playground. Kenny said the boys called him "hyper" and told him to go take another "hyper pill." When she prodded a little more, her son admitted it was hard for him to keep his eye on the ball and his mind on the outfield. She explained why this was difficult and that the medication might help with this problem. A few days later Kenny told his mom how when he told some friends that he had a concentration problem and wasn't an airhead, they didn't tease him at all.

Explain How Medication May Help.

Your child probably has a fairly sophisticated history of experiences with other medications. She is likely to have used several kinds of antibiotics, pain medications, fever reducers, salves, ointments, cough syrups, and other medicines. Your child is also likely to know someone who wears glasses, uses knee braces, or has a hearing aid. You can use your child's understanding of medical treatment to explain the decision to try medication.

Older youngsters and adolescents may want to understand more about the reasons they have difficulty paying attention and concentrating, but it is important for all children to understand that any of the medications used to treat ADHD do not cure the problem. Unlike antibiotics or other medications with which they might be familiar, ADHD medications do not "fight" and "kill" bacteria or swiftly vanquish a cough or an earache. Instead, they work with the brain to help a person gain control over some aspect of behavior. They are "helpers." You might use the "eyeglasses" analogy: Just as eyeglasses help a child to see better, medications may help a child pay attention better, sit still more easily, and concentrate better. And just as eyeglasses will not read for a child, medications cannot learn or do the work for a child. That is up to her.

Motivate Your Child to Cope.

Your goal is to work positively with your child to cope with different aspects of ADHD and to improve performance. When you do make a match with the right medication, both you and your child are likely to feel more ready to try new approaches to deal with various facets of the disorder.

In addition, your explanation of ADHD can help your child see in a new light the characteristics that are troublesome. For example, rather than being described as "distractible," a young man was told he just noticed everything. That was great in some situations, because he was so observant. However, he learned he had to control his attention in other situations, because noticing everything could be a hindrance.

Inform Your Child That You Are Going to Explain the Problem to Siblings, Grandparents, Teachers, and Other Important People in the Child's Life.

ADHD children do not live in a vacuum. Their troubling behaviors can spill over into all kinds of relationships. Enlisting these significant people on the child's support team can only be helpful in the long run.

ADHD is especially hard on siblings. Although they might not have the deficit, they often experience the brunt of the situation. Many siblings are embarrassed by their brother or sister's behavior. They may also be jealous of all the special attention the ADHD sibling seems to get. Use the same type of guidelines to explain ADHD to siblings, and then make sure you give them time to express their feelings, ask questions, and understand what you are trying to do. There are a number of books you can read with siblings to help in this process. *My Brother's a World-Class Pain* by Dr. Michael Gordon is one such book.

Grandparents often have difficulty understanding ADHD. If they live far away, they may be unaware of some of the behaviors that distress you. Or, not being familiar with the disorder, they may simply assume that some old-fashioned discipline would resolve the problem. Explain the disorder and what you are doing to help the child so that grandparents can support your efforts.

GETTING STARTED ON MEDICATION

Most stimulant medications are initially prescribed in the short-acting form, given before school and perhaps at lunchtime. Close monitoring of the child's behavior provides important information on which to base decisions about medication.

The optimum situation for determining the effectiveness of medication is a double-blind placebo-controlled test. No one—not the child, the parent or the teacher—knows when the child is on medication or placebo. However, most often, professionals have neither access to placebos nor time to conduct such a test. Having a treatment team, including the child, parent, physician, psychologist, and possibly other professionals, to provide feedback about performance on and off medication is an excellent alternative.

MONITORING MEASURES

You are probably quite familiar with one tool for monitoring behavior: the types of measures used when the diagnosis of ADHD was made. Those same behavior checklists and longer parent and teacher questionnaires can provide new insight about your own or your child's behavior. In addition, a home-school feedback system can give you daily or weekly information about behavior. (See Chapters 3 and 4.)

When medication is administered, shorter forms of parent and teacher questionnaires can provide ongoing information that aids the physician in determining optimum medication level and designing other forms of treatment. For example, the shorter form of the Conners Teacher Rating Scale can be used to determine if adjustments to medication dosages are indicated. Positive changes in behavior might indicate that the dosage is moving toward the right level, whereas negative changes in behavior indicate that adjustments are needed.

We have found that a crucial element of successful monitoring is how easy the tool is to use. If the system is too complicated or time-consuming, no one, no matter how diligent, will continue to use it for very long. Simple, quick, easy-to-understand feedback reports provide valuable daily information about a child's attention and activity level in school.

Each day or in each class, the teacher simply marks the amount of work completed and the individual's activity level. The Daily Report on page 76 in Chapter 4 is better suited for the younger child, while the Summary Report on page 77 will be less embarrassing for an older child or adolescent.

SCHEDULING MEDICATION

Most people assume that medication should be given at a particular time, usually before a child goes to school and at noon. However, just as there are individual responses to medication, the timing of medication should also be individualized to fit each person's schedule and needs. Some children resent taking medication at school. Another child's schedule may be such that he would be better served by taking his stimulant medication an hour later or after he gets to school so that its effects will peak later in the morning when subject demands are greater.

Fourteen-year-old Jocelyn found that she could manage homeroom and first-period art class quite well, but needed her Ritalin to peak later in the morning so she could cope with the demands of French and math class. Her lunch period was at 1:00 P.M., which allowed her to easily take a second dose of Ritalin at 1:30 P.M.

It's usually fairly easy to adjust the timing of some medications. Of course, longer-lasting timed-release forms of medication often help alleviate these concerns.

A NOT-SO-FINAL WORD ABOUT USING MEDICATION

Medication is never the first choice of treatment for ADHD. Perhaps even more important, medication should never be considered the last choice of treatment. Medication is only a part of the treatment for ADHD. This will become increasingly clear as you understand what medication can and cannot do for ADHD. Chapters 6 through 12 present in detail the facts about how medication influences self-control, learning, attention, social skills, organization, and other aspects of ADHD.

6

WHY ON-TASK IN THE CLASSROOM IS NOT ENOUGH

Improving Learning and Achievement

In elementary school, JACK *showed many characteristics of ADHD. He was not overly active, but he tended to get distracted easily, had a short attention span, and appeared to be very forgetful. His teacher said he often didn't have his homework done, did not complete seat work, and frequently didn't attend to what was happening in class. At home, his behavior was not a problem, although his parents often served as his memory and had to supervise his getting dressed and completing many daily tasks.*

When Jack was placed on medication, he seemed to undergo an amazing transformation. He completed his work on time, and his attention span for learning seemed to have doubled. His grades improved, and he seemed to feel much better about himself.

Unfortunately, by the time Jack got to middle school, everyone was shocked to find that his scores on standardized achievement tests had dropped considerably. Despite all the work he had done, he was several years behind in a number of subject areas. His parents began receiving reports that he did not complete homework assignments, and his grades began to fall. At home, Jack became moody and downright angry. He would blow up over the least-expected things. He needed both special-educational help and therapy.

If your child were not having problems in the classroom, there's a good chance that she would not have been diagnosed with attention deficit hyperactivity disorder. You wouldn't be considering medication; you might not even be reading this book.

Why do we make such strong, definite statements? First of all, many young children's troublesome behavior is written off to immaturity or "being all boy" (or tomboy) until they get to school. Young children are not supposed to be able to sit still; they naturally have short attention spans. If you are not a child-development expert or an experienced parent, you may not be aware that a young child's behavior is unusual or extreme. In fact, until your child is required to pay attention and sit for periods of the day—usually in first grade—no one with whom your child has had prolonged contact may have the range of experience to note that a particular behavior is unusual or out-of-bounds. Furthermore, many children who are not hyperactive but who have difficulty concentrating and paying attention are not diagnosed until their difficulties in learning become apparent in school.

A great portion of the controversy about ADHD children and the distrust of medication for them stems from many parents' belief that teachers and school administrators are too quick to recommend medication for a child who exhibits ADHD-like behaviors, and that they do so simply to keep him or her under control. The media have also been swift to report evidence to support such a notion. A series of articles published in 1987, in newspapers across the country including *The New York Times*, described sharp increases in the sales of Ritalin and questioned whether the medication was being prescribed "unusually often" in some states. Again in 1987, the American Academy of Pediatrics urged pediatricians to use caution in prescribing medication for this disorder. However, in reality, the rate of increase in prescribing Ritalin matches the trend-analysis data used by the Drug Enforcement Administration to determine production quotas of Ritalin and the Food and Drug Administration's estimate of medical need for methylphenidate. Given the estimates of the number of school-age children who are affected by ADHD, as discussed in Chapter 2, the use of medication in most schools does not appear to be excessive.

EFFECTS OF ADHD ON STUDENTS IN THE CLASSROOM

ADHD places those who have it in great jeopardy in school. In the regular classroom, ADHD youngsters face a risk of failure two to three times greater than that of their peers. They are more likely to receive lower grades in academics and score lower on achievement tests in math and reading. They are likely to be one to two years behind in math, reading, spelling, and language. Drs. Weiss and Hechtman, in the retrospective studies of ADHD children grown up, found that one third of them failed to graduate from high school. These are alarming numbers.

WHAT MEDICATION CAN DO

In this chapter, we will review what medication does and doesn't do for those ADHD students who are responders and what else you must do to help the ADHD child succeed in the classroom. Understanding the effects of medication on classroom behavior will give you a handle on your child's learning experience so that you can determine what other kinds of interventions and experiences will help your child succeed in the classroom.

One thing is clear: We don't know a lot about how medication affects academic knowledge. Most findings relate to academic performance *in the laboratory, not in the classroom.* Most studies have been completed in laboratory settings using tests such as the Paired Associates Learning Tests (PALT) and the Continuous Performance Test (CPT) that normally would not be found in the classroom. Nor have the results, although valuable and interesting, been shown to predict a student's response to medication in the classroom. Also keep in mind that most of the studies that have been done on the effects of medication on academic learning involve stimulant medication, most often Ritalin.

Since each child's individual response to medication is unique, the only true means to determine the effects of a particular dosage of medication on a particular type of task is to monitor a child's performance in the classroom. Your child's experience with medication, no matter how good, is likely to help him in specific ways that can be determined only by observation.

Having said all that, there are some things we do know about the general effects of medication on an ADHD child's classroom performance. Clearly, medication does make some important differences in the classroom for children who respond to it.

1. Children May Complete More Work.
A number of studies have shown that methylphenidate increases student productivity. For example, in terms of arithmetic performance, ADHD students on medication generally will attempt more problems, and also solve more problems.

2. Students' Work Is Often More Accurate.

Not only will they complete more problems, the number of correct answers also increases. On the basis of their research, Drs. Pelham and Milich from Western Psychiatric Institute and the University of Kentucky, respectively, suggest that a student taking medication might increase production on arithmetic problems by as much as 30 percent with no loss of accuracy. Unfortunately, as we implied previously, there is no clear answer to the question, "What dose of medication will provide optimal arithmetic performance for the average ADHD child?" The only way to determine the efficacy of medication for a particular child is to carefully observe and monitor that child's performance and adjust dosages accordingly.

3. ADHD Students on Medication Are Often "On-Task" More.

That means they are doing the requested task as requested with less off-task behavior. It's not simply a matter of doing more work more quickly. The students appear to be on-task for longer periods of time. Since they are off-task for less time, the effort is more consistent.

4. It's Harder to Tell the ADHD Students from Their Peers.

Observing in the classroom, it's more difficult to distinguish ADHD children on medication from their classmates. That's a very positive finding. Dr. Howard Abikoff, from Long Island Jewish Hillside Medical Center, and Dr. Rachel Gittelman, of New York State Psychiatric Institute, as long ago as 1985, found that methylphenidate "normalized" the behavior of ADHD children in a number of ways. Before treatment, the twenty-eight children studied were conspicuous in the time spent out of their seats, the amount of small motor movements, calling out and solicitation of the teacher, noncompliance with teachers' requests, and overall hyperactivity. While on medication, the same students were significantly improved in all measures except attentiveness. In fact, in many ways, the ADHD students were indistinguishable from their peers who were not ADHD.

5. Medication May Improve Short-Term Performance.

For many of the reasons listed, daily performance is better for children on medication. That makes sense. They are on-task more often, paying better attention to the teacher, and doing better work in the classroom. That makes everyone happier, and at least in the short run, these students are less distinguishable from their classmates, and their classroom performance is more like their peers'.

6. Medication May Improve Inattentive Students' Grades.

At least for students who are diagnosed as having an attention deficit primarily inattentive type, there is some justification for expecting grades to improve. In a study of ten students conducted by Drs. Richard Famularo and Terence Fenton of Harvard Medical School, the children's letter grades during and for the period after drug treatment showed significant improvement in at least three of five subject areas.

7. Medication Affects Various Kinds of Learning Differently.

Although there has been much discussion that greater doses of Ritalin may actually impair learning, Dr. Mary Solanto, of the Albert Einstein College of Medicine, did not find this to be true from her review of the research literature. However, the research does show that there is great variability among children's responses to medication, and that the particular dose of medication that maximizes performance in one area may not be the same dosage to maximize performance in another area of learning.

Other studies indicate children's memory for visual information improves on medication. This is especially true of short-term recall of visual stimuli.

8. Students' Behavior Ratings May Improve.

Teacher ratings of children who respond well to medication often reflect a remarkable improvement in behavior. In general, children are more compliant, show less extraneous movement, and engage in fewer aggressive-type behaviors both in the classroom and on the playground.

9. Students Often Appear Less Frustrated.

Some studies indicate a positive effect in that children on medication are able to persevere in the face of frustrating tasks. ADHD children are often easily frustrated and get angry with a task. On medication these children are able to inhibit those impulses and continue a challenging task for longer periods of time.

10. Students' Quiz and Test Scores May Show Improvement.

Although there is no indication that achievement-test scores improve as a result of taking medication, in the short run older students show improved quiz and test scores and greater attention to classwork, including seat work and teacher lectures. Research that shows improvement in learning has utilized teacher-designed written tasks to measure academic performance.

WHAT MEDICATION CANNOT DO

Unfortunately, medication does not solve all the learning problems for individuals with ADHD. As one ADHD adult told us, "Now that I understand what ADHD is and have seen the differences medication can make, Ritalin would have helped me. But I still would have had to work like . . ."

1. Students on Medication Do Not Show Long-Term Improvement on Achievement Tests.

This continues to be a major disappointment. Despite the fact that medication improves productivity and performance, a student's knowledge over time has not been shown to increase. For example, although children do more math problems with greater accuracy, there is no indication that this reflects an increased mastery of math. It doesn't make sense. They are doing more work, paying better attention to their teachers, and performing better in the classroom.

There are a number of possible explanations for this phenomenon. The simplest and most compelling is that perhaps achievement tests and intelligence tests are the wrong measure to track short-term learning. In addition, such tests may not reflect the actual teaching and learning taking place in the classroom. Achievement tests typically have only one or two items on a particular aspect of a subject, although a number of weeks of class time may have been spent on that topic. Finally, the stagnant format of most achievement tests does not permit a student to interact with the material and to show a variety of responses.

2. Effects of Medication on Cognitive Functioning Vary.

There is some indication that the effects of medication on a particular area of function vary across doses and across individuals. We've said repeatedly that medication affects each student differently. In addition, it appears what may be good for one type of academic performance may not be good for another. For example, a student's accuracy in completing math calculations may improve, but his performance on word problems may decrease when he is on medication.

3. Medication Does Not Teach Unmastered Academic Skills or Fill Gaps in Learning.

This is another "big one." No ADHD medication can put knowledge into your child's head. On medication or off, she can't do what she doesn't know how to do. If she didn't know how to divide decimals before going on medication, she still won't know how to do it on medication. The key difference is that she is likely to be more receptive to the material being presented.

4. Some Investigations Have Failed to Show Any Positive Effects of Medication for Primarily Learning-Disabled Children.

Children whose ADHD is complicated by additional problems may not experience as great a positive change on medication. Medication will not correct basic processing problems. However, conventional wisdom would indicate that if medication improves attention, children with ADHD plus a learning disability who respond to medication should be more receptive to the specialized instruction that will help them overcome their learning difficulties.

QUESTIONS TO ASK ABOUT YOUR STUDENT

Medication for ADHD will not solve your child's learning problems. Numerous studies have shown that children on medication for ADHD experience short-term improvements in behavior, academics, and social interactions. However, as the previous summary noted, research findings do not indicate that medication brings about long-term academic achievement. In addition, many of the problems that children have off medication in the classroom, especially those directly related to the mastery of particular academic skills, remain.

What does this mean? On a day-to-day basis, if your child is a responder to medication, her behavior and attentiveness in the classroom are bound to improve—perhaps dramatically. In fact, if your child is diagnosed as ADHD very early on and her problems in the classroom relate more to behavior than to learning, there is a chance that medication may almost *appear* to be a miracle cure.

The more common scenario has fewer elements of surprise. Your child on medication is likely to be more attentive to teacher requests. An observer in the classroom may have difficulty identifying your child as the one with ADHD, because she will be less disruptive and will be on-task doing the assigned work more of the time. In addition, her class work is likely to be completed more quickly and accurately than previously. Her handwriting and the neatness of her papers might also improve, as might daily quiz and test scores.

On the downside, for most ADHD students, medication will not eradicate all problems in the classroom, and additional interventions will be needed.

Why is this true? If children are more attentive on a daily basis, shouldn't they also do better in school? It comes down to this: Being on-task in the classroom is not enough. At the very least, there are three problems that influence your child's improved achievement in the classroom.

1. Does Your Child Have Additional Learning Problems That Affect His Knowledge or Performance in the Classroom?

Approximately one third of children with ADHD also have learning disabilities. These learning difficulties may affect the way your child is able to receive, assimilate, or express information. For example, a child may have normal visual acuity, yet have difficulty discriminating similar letters or words, making it difficult for him to learn to read. Another child may easily perceive visual stimuli, yet have short- or long-term memory problems that make it difficult for him to retain the information he is taught. And still another student may have expressive language problems, so that although she knows the answer to a question, she has great difficulty putting the answer into words either orally or in writing. If your child has basic information-processing problems, he will still have them on medication.

2. Does Your Child Have Deficits in Knowledge or Skills That Will Make It Difficult for Him to Learn?

Depending on how long your child has had difficulties in school, he is bound to have gaps in learning that will affect the assimilation of new information. If you don't have the prerequisite information for a task, it will be very difficult to succeed. No matter how well your child pays attention, if he is missing some core skill or information—such as the arithmetic mastery needed to tackle algebra, or the spelling and grammar skills required for writing—he is unlikely to succeed.

3. Does Your Child Have a History of Experience That Leads to a Defeatist Attitude?

It's misleading to simply state, "Most ADHD students are under-achievers." Underachieving implies the student is not working up to his potential. We don't know what your child's potential is, but there is a good chance it is hard for him to keep up, hard to keep track of things, hard to cover up. It's just downright hard to be ADHD in the fast-moving, demanding environments most children and adolescents travel in. Your child may work very hard in the classroom yet always feel his best is not good enough. If your child has a history of failure in the classroom, no amount of medication will erase those memories, or the feelings they prompt, overnight.

Perseverance and attitude are affected by self-concept. Learning to believe "I can do this" will take time. Not only may there be skills your child missed, there are also new risks your child must learn to take. If he failed repeatedly before, it will take a little longer for him to take the risk of failure again.

WHAT ELSE YOU MUST DO TO HELP YOUR CHILD SUCCEED IN SCHOOL

Research indicates that a *combination of medication and educational and behavioral interventions* are often needed to maximize the ADHD student's learning.

Medications appear to have greater behavior-changing effects when combined with other effective treatment approaches. Think of it this way: Medication is best seen as an *enabler*. For those students, elementary-age or older, who respond positively, medication allows them to be better able to approach the learning task. They can attend better, control motion, be less impulsive, and respond more appropriately to teacher's requests. They will still need additional help both in and out of the classroom to reach their potential for learning.

PROVIDE OPTIMAL STRUCTURE AND FEEDBACK

As outlined previously, providing optimal instruction for ADHD youth is often a matter of manipulating elements of the environment, adapting materials, and changing the way the teacher works with the child. Findings in the research point to a number of principles to keep in mind when working with ADHD students. Earlier, in Chapter 4, we detailed several of these techniques as alternatives to taking medication (see the cross-referenced pages following). If medication is deemed necessary, the eight principles below *are strongly recommended* here as crucial components of an effective overall treatment program.

Principle #1: Manipulate the learning environment to increase small group interactions with the teacher and increase the ability of the teacher to monitor individual students' behavior (pages 61–64).

Gaining and maintaining the ADHD child's attention to a task is crucial. Medication helps with this. So does setting up an environment that will increase the percentage of time the child is engaged in direct learning in the classroom.

ADHD children respond best to one-on-one supervision. Learning situations in which a small number of students work directly with a teacher improve the ADHD child's attention and on-task behavior. The chances that a student will follow through on a command are increased when the child's behavior is supervised immediately following the instruction given.

Principle #2: Find the optimal seat in the classroom and/or change the classroom setting (see page 58).

As discussed in Chapter 4, several studies and a great deal of teacher experience indicate that classroom seating has an impact on children's tendency to pay attention. This is especially true of ADHD youth. For example, seating that facilitates social interaction may be good for discussion but impedes on-task behavior. When a child's seat provides for optimum teacher supervision with minimal distraction, on-task behavior may improve significantly. However, there are times when the best placement for an ADHD child is a specialized classroom with a low student-teacher ratio and individualized instruction.

The best seat in a classroom for your child is likely to change from subject to subject and teacher to teacher. The teacher's instructional style and the type of tasks will influence where the best seat might be.

Mrs. Ward teaches sixth-grade literature. Half of the class period is spent in independent reading time, during which Mrs. Ward calls individual students for appointments at her desk. For a good portion of the rest of the time, individual students come to the teacher's desk with questions. Placing an ADHD student next to her desk does allow Mrs. Ward to monitor the student, but it also places the student in the line of a continuously changing flow of students to the teacher's desk.

Principle #3: Provide opportunities for the ADHD student to give and receive feedback about what he is working on in the classroom (see page 61).

The elements of good instruction are the same for everyone. Good teaching involves presenting specific information through a sequence of activities designed to facilitate learning by providing opportunities for practice, feedback, and the chance to apply the new learning in a variety of situations over time. The chance to get additional feedback and review should be built into the system.

Some students will learn no matter how the material is presented. However, all of the elements of good instruction are probably more crucial to the success of the ADHD student or one with learning difficulties. In a typical situation, a teacher gives directions and the class begins working—all except the ADHD student, that is. His mind was elsewhere when the directions were given, or he heard only part of the teacher's request. Students with ADHD benefit from the simple opportunity to repeat the instructions or restate the purpose of a task, prior to starting. The feedback loop is crucial to the ADHD student.

Principle #4: Use positive and negative consequences to improve student on-task behaviors and rule-following in the classroom (see pages 69–70).

The majority of ADHD students are underachievers because they fail to complete assignments, fail to accurately complete written tasks and tests, and/or are inattentive when learning is presented. Many people have found that behavior management, either alone or combined with medication, can improve ADHD children's in-class behavior. Research indicates that behavior management focusing on positive reinforcement, negative consequences, and response costs can be effective in reducing disruptive behavior and increasing attentiveness to tasks. A number of studies have proven the effectiveness of praise and positive reinforcement in increasing attentiveness and on-task behaviors in ADHD students. Specifically, Ayllon, Layman, and Kandel of Georgia State University found that reinforcement of academic performance suppressed hyperactivity and improved on-task behavior in the classroom. When students were reinforced with a point system for work completed, reading and math performance dramatically increased.

For some individuals, however, praise is simply not a strong enough motivator to maintain on-task behavior. In fact, most research indicates that ADHD students need both positive and negative consequences built into any behavioral management system for optimum results. A token system in which students are awarded points for appropriate behavior, and are sanctioned with negative consequences following inappropriate behavior, can be very successful (see pages 73–74). Negative consequences may take the form of response cost in which the student loses privileges, tokens or points when he fails to meet a particular work criteria or displays inappropriate behavior. Other negative consequences often effectively used in the classroom to promote appropriate behavior include time-out (see pages 70–72). Time-out from positive reinforcement is given for short periods of time as a consequence of inappropriate behavior. For example, a child might be excluded from receiving points for five minutes in response to interrupting the classroom. Time-out may be applied by physically excluding a child from a group by placing him in a chair away from peers, by using a time-out card placed on the child's desk, or by symbolically enforcing time-out with a ribbon tied on a young child's hand.

Principle #5: Use a home-school feedback system to reinforce academics and appropriate classroom behavior (see pages 74–76).

Home-school contingency systems have been shown to be very effective for ADHD children. Such systems have the advantage of including parents in the information loop. This can be especially effective for a teacher who is reluctant to alter her teaching style for the ADHD student. In that case, a checklist or chart system that monitors student behavior is superimposed on the normal school day so that the parent can reinforce the child for completing assignments or controlling behavior. See Chapter 4 for details on how to implement a home-school report that will track target behaviors on a daily or weekly basis.

Principle #6: Provide a structured classroom with rules to promote appropriate behavior and increased on-task behavior (see pages 61–63).

At the minimum, ADHD youth function best in well-structured settings. They need to know what is expected of them in both daily activities and behavior. A daily schedule should be presented in a concrete manner using a calendar or clock as a reference. Changes in the schedule should be clearly announced.

Class rules should also be clearly displayed. Taught specifically through role-playing and other approaches, the rules should be posted and retaught frequently. When children are following the rules, that should be noted. Infractions of the rules should be clearly defined and consequences applied.

Principle #7: Modify the length and form of assignments (see pages 65–67).

It is crucial to recognize that for the ADHD student, working for long periods of time unsupervised may result in greater off-task behavior. Children may be discouraged by a number of assignments presented simultaneously. In addition, since these children often have difficulty with fine-motor skills, copying board work can present a unique problem for them. In general, ADHD children will perform better on short assignments, with decreased writing. Copying from a paper, using the computer, and using manipulatives or creative oral and artistic means to express ideas are other ways to spur the child to show his knowledge.

In addition, any intervention that organizes the student's work effort or materials can improve performance. Breaking tasks into manageable pieces, reinforcing work done in small time frames, or prompting particular behaviors can be successful. Chapter 9, "Routines Medication Does Not Teach," discusses this concept in detail.

Principle #8: Use instructional materials that focus the student's selective attention (see pages 65–68).

Part of the difficulty for ADHD children in completing independent assignments is that they do not automatically know what to attend to. Although most people consider this a problem of an attention deficit, some researchers view the problem as one of *attentional bias,* in that children are prone to attend to particular types of stimuli, regardless of prevailing need. Even though medication improves the ability to attend, these youngsters are not automatically aware of what they should focus on—at least for the purposes of instruction.

In general, most children thrive in a classroom where instructional strategies and materials match their interests and abilities. An enthusiastic, knowledgeable teacher can use novelty—such as changes in color, shape, and design—to capture the attention of students. Students are much less likely to become bored if tasks and assignments vary in type and length, format and color. Also, activities that vary from sedentary to active are more likely to maintain a child's attention.

FILL IN ACADEMIC GAPS

Often by the time ADHD has been diagnosed, many students have already developed large gaps in their knowledge or have missed certain skills. No matter how hard a student tries or how well he can pay attention on medication, unless these learning deficits are filled, there is no way he can succeed. Like a snowball rolling downhill, the learning deficit continues to grow unless it is addressed.

The deficit may be in a particular subject area such as math or reading, where learning is cumulative and one skill forms the foundation for the next. If you do not know your multiplication facts, it will be almost impossible to learn division.

Or gaps in one subject area may affect skills in another area. When a student is unable to concentrate in order to develop reading skills, writing and spelling are affected, and the acquisition of knowledge through reading for all subjects is thwarted.

An educational evaluation will determine whether an individual has learning deficits. Since ADHD students often do not do well on group-administered tests, individual testing is advised. Your school system may conduct an individual assessment, or you may need to use the services of a professional outside the system to administer individual tests in a private setting.

Once you have pinpointed the areas of deficit, it is likely you will need specialized help. If the knowledge gap is great enough, your youngster may qualify for special programming in math, reading, or other areas. Since many ADHD youth enjoy using the computer, your youngster may benefit from computerized programs available for drill and practice in subjects like math and reading.

For many students, learning comes most easily through one-to-one instruction. If you are able to employ a specialized tutor, you or your child may find that learning is more rapid.

TEACH STUDY SKILLS AND TEST-TAKING SKILLS

In addition to needing assistance in specific subject areas, many people with ADHD need help with study skills. Learning how to learn is just as important as acquiring information.

Many ADHD students do not know how to change their study habits to meet the special needs of various subject areas. Often they are unable to systematically divide material into manageable pieces to study efficiently.

There are a number of instructional techniques that may improve the ADHD student's studying ability. Using a study-skills approach can provide the student with a systematic means to read and learn material without straining attention. For example, SQ3R teaches a student to *Sur*vey and pose *Q*uestions about the material before *R*eading and then to *R*eview and *R*ecite information after reading, Learning how to take notes, underline efficiently, and outline material also increases effective study time and learning ability.

All the studying in the world is not sufficient if the student does not know how to take a test. Many ADHD students cannot produce information on demand. Others do not understand how to answer true-false questions or how to complete an essay test. Becoming sophisticated in learning how to take various kinds of tests will help the student score better on exams. In fact, it may be a weakness in test-taking skills that hinders the ADHD student's performance on standardized achievement tests, including college entrance exams.

There are a number of courses available for learning study skills and test-taking strategies. However, ADHD individuals often learn such skills more quickly in a one-to-one setting. No matter what your age, don't be embarrassed by needing a tutor. Adults often hire "consultants" to help us with all types of problems, and even the most intellectually gifted students turn to special "test-taking" courses for college and postgraduate test training.

GET SPECIAL HELP FOR LEARNING DISABILITIES

It is estimated that one third of ADHD students have a learning disability or significant processing problem. Such a disability or problem places additional strains on attention. Students who are both ADHD and LD learn differently and need specialized educational help to progress. They must learn how to use their strengths to compensate for areas of weakness. Typically, students with learning disabilities require specialized instruction from trained people.

In order for your child to be eligible for special help for learning disabilities, additional testing to validate the existence of LD and ADHD will be necessary. Once testing is completed, you may request a "staffing" at your child's school to review the results. During this meeting an individual educational plan, or IEP, will be developed, educational goals will be defined, and eligibility for the services needed to reach these goals will be determined. As a parent of a child with ADHD and learning disabilities, you should be aware that your child is eligible for assistance as defined by Public Law 94-142. Ask the school for a brochure that explains these rights.

Staffings should be cooperative ventures between parents and school personnel. However, schools have limited resources. You may want to supplement your child's instruction with help from a trained learning specialist outside the school system, if you can afford it. Joining groups like the Learning Disabilities Association of America (LDA) and Children with Attention Deficit Disorder (Ch.A.D.D.) can provide you with additional information and support to meet your needs.

GET SPECIAL PERMISSION TO TAKE STANDARDIZED TESTS DIFFERENTLY

Many students with ADHD do not do well on standardized tests given under standard conditions. Anyone with a documented diagnosis of ADHD can qualify to take many standardized exams, such as college entrance examinations, under special conditions: for example, with extended time limits or in a quieter setting with fewer distractions. If the student has a learning disability, you may also request additional accommodations. To qualify, you must have a letter from the psychologist or other specialist who did the original testing for ADHD or made the diagnosis.

WORK WITH THE SYSTEM

As your youngster moves through the educational system, you may find there are more or fewer adjustments to be made. You should work toward your student's acquiring such a level of sophistication in managing the symptoms of ADHD that he becomes his own best advocate with teachers and administrators.

Understanding the differing expectations of teachers, the student may find an advantage to being able to select at least part of his own curriculum in high school. He may also find alternative ways of taking notes and completing written assignments. We have known students who were allowed to take laptop computers to class and even take tests on the computer. Others have been allowed to copy classmates' notes on a regular basis and check assignments with a study buddy. The more the student explains to his teachers about ADHD, the more likely he will be to get the help he needs.

Getting ready for college is a challenging, stressful period for all students. Many students find they are more comfortable and achieve well at a small college with a strong element of special programming for ADHD and learning-disabled students. Be sure to work with a counselor who is knowledgeable about colleges with specialized programs and support for ADHD and learning-disabled students. Fortunately, today there are increasing numbers of colleges that have such programs. An excellent source of information about getting ready for college is *ADD and the College Student*, by Patricia O. Quinn, M.D.

A FINAL WORD ABOUT ACHIEVEMENT

Your child may be one of the few for whom medication makes such a drastic and positive change in the classroom that little else is necessary for success. But don't expect that to happen. For most students, even those who respond to medication, improvements in attention and behavior are only the first steps to achieving up to potential. Further instructional programming and help are needed to allow ADHD students to maneuver in the learning environment in a productive manner. The need for help continues even into the college years.

As an adult, you may find that the diagnosis of ADHD frees

you to seek the kind of help that did not exist when you were in school. You may discover that years of failure can be undone by new techniques and the support of trained professionals who understand the special conditions you must work through. It is never too late to learn.

7

THE MISCUE DILEMMA

Solving Social Problems

Eight-year-old ALAN *is an active child who seems to be in continuous motion. With his reputation preceding him, he is quickly labeled the class clown year after year. He gets a lot of attention in the classroom, but what he would rather have are friends. At recess, he watches the boys play four square, not knowing how to join the game. At other times he blurts out his opinion and offends classmates. He's totally unaware of the looks that pass among the kids when he drops his books, yells out an answer, or takes over a discussion.*

BONNIE *is a quiet fifteen-year-old. She doesn't get into trouble, but has always had difficulty keeping up in school. She is always on the sidelines, and friendships come and go. Her parents fear that her desire to fit in and make friends might lead her to join the wrong crowd.*

Twenty-four-year-old BRUCE *is a computer programmer. Programming fits his style. As he says, he likes software better than people. His coworkers believe that to be true. They say he's rude, leaves without talking, and never shows any interest in what they're doing. He says they're boring. Bruce has been divorced once, has two children, and is worried his second marriage is on the skids. His wife says she can't stand his unpredictability or the piles of mess that accompany his presence.*

Although each of these individuals is very different, they have some things in common. They have all been diagnosed as ADHD, and they are all struggling to handle their daily schedules and find a place in the world. More often than not, though, their actions alienate them from their peers. Unfortunately, Alan, Bonnie, and Bruce are often unaware of the negative response many of their actions draw. Furthermore, Bruce's history of feeling like an outsider has turned him against his peers, so he has accepted his role as a loner.

How do you help ADHD children make and keep friends? How do you prevent impulsive ADHD teenagers from making the wrong friends? How do you help ADHD adults avoid missing social cues and maintain lasting relationships? Does taking medication solve the problems ADHD youth and adults have in getting along with others?

WHAT'S YOUR CHILD'S OR YOUR OWN SOCIAL QUOTIENT?

Some people seem to automatically know how to behave in various situations. We say they have a high SQ, or social quotient. They seem to be aware of others' actions and are very sensitive to the feelings of the people around them. It is almost as though they anticipate what their friends and acquaintances are thinking. At the very least, they always seem to do and say exactly the right thing.

What is your child's SQ? How about your own? Answer each question in Table 7.1 with a *Y* for yes if the answer is true for you or your child most of the time, and an *N* for no if the answer is not true for you or your child most of the time. It might be interesting to verify your views by having your spouse or a friend also complete the survey for you or your child.

Table 7.1

What's Your Social Quotient?

Answer each question with a Y for yes if it is true most of the time, or an N for no if it is not true most of the time for you or your child. Place your answer in the box provided in either column.

CONVERSATION SKILLS
1. Do you enjoy being around peers?
2. Are you often bored when talking with others?
3. Do you use a pleasant face and voice when you speak to others?

☐ 4. Do you find yourself looking away from the person you are speaking to?

☐ 5. Do you make and keep eye contact with the person you are talking to?

☐ 6. Do you touch the person you are talking to?

☐ 7. Do you greet someone with a positive hello?

☐ 8. Do you find yourself wiggling or swaying or needing to move when you are having a conversation?

☐ 9. Do you maintain a comfortable physical distance between yourself and others?

☐ 10. Do you change topics a lot when talking to others?

☐ 11. Do you know how to start a conversation?

☐ 12. Do you tend to dominate a conversation?

☐ 13. Can you keep a conversation going?

☐ 14. Do you find yourself in a group and not know what to say to the person next to you?

☐ 15. Are you interested in what others have to say?

☐ 16. Do you find it difficult to talk about one topic?

☐ 17. Do you compliment others?

☐ 18. Do you get impatient waiting for your turn?

BUILDING RELATIONSHIPS

☐ 19. Do you share?

☐ 20. Do you dislike being told no for an answer?

☐ 21. Do you take the role of compromiser in a group?

☐ 22. Do you usually think it is someone else's fault when something goes wrong?

☐ 23. Do you accept responsibility for your own actions?

☐ 24. Do you want to hear how others feel?

☐ 25. Do you recognize when others are acting inappropriately?

☐ 26. Do you feel uncomfortable joining an activity in progress?

HANDLING EMOTIONS AND DIFFICULT SITUATIONS

☐ 27. Can you label what you are feeling?

☐ 28. Do you get angry quickly?

☐ 29. Can you express your feelings to others without getting angry?

☐ 30. Do you dislike unexpected occurrences?

☐ 31. Do you express your opinion so others want to listen?

☐ 32. Do you tend to barge into a situation without thinking?

☐ 33. Do you ask for help when you need it?

☐ 34. Do you get angry when you can't do something well?

☐ 35. Do you accept constructive criticism?

☐ 36. Do you have trouble accepting disappointment?

☐ **TOTAL Y RESPONSES**

☐ **TOTAL N RESPONSES**

CALCULATING YOUR OR YOUR CHILD'S SQ

Count up the number of Y's in the first column and put the total in the appropriate box at the bottom. Total the number of N's in the second column and place that number in the box at the bottom.

A perfect score would be 18 yeses in the first column and 18 noes in the second column. Of course, no one is perfect or "perfectly social." The higher the number of yeses in column one and noes in column two, the more socially astute you are.

Look at the odd-numbered questions. Which ones did you answer no to? Review the even-numbered questions. Which ones did you answer yes to? These items provide clues to the types of social skills you or your child will need to work on.

If you or your child has scores that indicate less social awareness and comfort, then your child's (or your own) social behavior may be interfering with positive interactions with friends.

ADHD AFFECTS ALL ASPECTS OF LIFE

Many parents assume that ADHD is something that affects children only in the classroom, so they don't give their children medication in the afternoon or on weekends. In response to a survey we conducted on an ADHD bulletin board on the Internet, one parent typed: "His teachers see the problems much more than we do, so we do not give him medication on weekends or in the summer." However, this same parent also indicated that homework and friendships—the pursuits he attempted without medication—were problem areas for her son.

Sometimes parents don't recognize the effects of ADHD outside the classroom. They make the mistake of assuming that the demands on attention are much greater and more important in the classroom than they are at home or at play. This is especially true when a child is not hyperactive or difficult to manage. Then they may overlook the effects of inattention in social interactions and simply label the child as shy. In a desire to lessen the child's time on medication, parents may be compounding the problem by withholding medication at the very times children are most likely to play with friends and siblings: after school, on weekends, and during holidays and vacations.

You have observed some of the difficulties your child has with other children. Certainly with siblings you may have noted the differences in children's reactions. Daily routines such as going to bed, getting dressed, and brushing teeth may move quite smoothly with one child in the family and be a lesson in willfulness with your ADHD child. The same problems that occur elsewhere arise at home only more often. Siblings may seem to spar constantly, so that you wonder if they will ever be friends. Although all siblings squabble, you may recognize a more troubling tone and degree to disagreements.

At school or during extracurricular activities, you may be able to arrange to observe your child from a window or some other unobtrusive location, so your presence goes unnoticed. It is an interesting and sometimes heartwrenching experience to watch an ADHD child on the playground. You are likely to see quick displays of temper, rapid mood swings, lack of attention to what's going on around him, and the tendency to blame others for problems. Or you may see your child standing on the sidelines, wanting to enter the mainstream but not knowing how.

Away from school, you may have listened as your child invited classmates over to play and hurt for him when he was turned down. Maybe you've watched from the stands as the ball whizzed past your child's glove because he was looking elsewhere, and then witnessed the jeering and teasing of his teammates. You may have felt his hurt when he was picked last for the team. As another father in our Internet survey typed, "I became the T-ball coach so my son wouldn't be kicked off the team, and I became the Cub Scout leader so he would be allowed to participate." If any of these situations rings true, the problem of what to do to help your child be socially successful is not lost on you.

As an ADHD adult, you may have felt yourself on the outside of a group and wondered how you got there. The sad part is that often even after you became an adolescent and more skilled at controlling your behavior, your peers remembered you the old way.

THE MISCUE DILEMMA

Children and adults who are popular with their peers appear to intuitively grasp how to make friends. This may be true. Research indicates that individuals who are more self-confident, outgoing, and supportive are better liked.

However, ADHD children whose attention flits here and there have an inherent problem: They easily miss crucial details of what's going on around them. Acting on "half the information," their reactions are sometimes out of sync with the rest of the group. We call this making a "miscue."

ADHD YOUTH AND ADULTS ARE SOMETIMES PERCEIVED AS BEING DIFFICULT

The aftereffects of such miscues is that ADHD youngsters are often perceived as being difficult and harder to get along with. Sometimes that's true. At other times, though, ADHD children and youth are at a total loss as to what they are doing wrong or why others don't seem to like them.

Medication can be helpful in social situations, but it is not the total answer. When old habits have been formed over a long time, ADHD youth must learn new behaviors before they can build new habits. The trouble is, your youngster may not have a clue as to what those new behaviors might be.

Carl clearly had this problem. Carl is a not terribly athletic child who had trouble maintaining his attention in the outfield. Ritalin helped him keep his eye on the ball, but it didn't help him learn to throw it. More important, if a teammate made a comment about an error he made, Carl didn't have the skills to shrug it off.

ADHD YOUTH DON'T RECOGNIZE HOW THEIR BEHAVIOR AFFECTS OTHERS

ADHD youth need help understanding how their behavior affects others and what it is they need to do instead. Inadvertently, without intending to offend anyone, ADHD individuals turn others off through small actions. For example, individuals with ADHD are more likely to change topics in the midst of a conversation and fail to listen to or look at others who are speaking. They may get up in the middle of a conversation or interrupt a speaker.

The very traits that characterize ADHD are in opposition to acting as part of a group. Acting impulsively, getting easily distracted, and not paying attention are behaviors that interfere with group dynamics. Being unable to take turns, displaying random outbursts, and being quick-tempered are characteristics that will not endear a child to his peers. Finally, add the fact that ADHD children do not "roll with the punches" and have difficulty making transitions from one activity to another.

In a nutshell, the social actions of ADHD children and youth are often off-base and way out of line. Unless they are playing video games all afternoon, classmates tire of catering to the erratic behavior of this friend and would prefer to play with someone else. Parents of classmates may prefer that their sons and daughters invite more agreeable and easier-to-manage children to play. They may even go so far as to discourage their own child from asking the ADHD youth to visit.

ADHD behavior often goes to extremes that make it difficult for everyone, including the ADHD youth or adult. No doubt you know that ADHD children are the kind of kids you want to hug at times for being so thoughtful. At other times, the force of their overreaction when something doesn't go their way or there is a change in plans leaves others shaking their heads in utter astonishment. It's not hard to understand why they encounter problems with making friends.

DEALING WITH EMOTIONS IS DIFFICULT FOR THE ADHD CHILD OR ADULT

Many ADHD adults and children hide their feelings; for others, emotions erupt like Mt. Vesuvius. As one set of parents remarked to us about their son, "We are always amazed when his teachers are surprised to learn Errol has a temper."

Perhaps no one outside the family can imagine your child has a temper either. But you've witnessed rip-roaring, wild displays of anger over an insignificant matter, the culmination of his having held it together all day at school. Then his temper recedes as rapidly as it appeared.

It's possible your child is like this, or these situations may be reminiscent of your own childhood, adolescence, and adulthood. Then again, maybe you have only heard the war stories of other parents about ADHD adolescents and adults, and now fear the difficulties that may lie ahead for your child and adolescent.

Building relationships, developing positive social skills, and solving problems take time to learn. Simply put, ADHD children need more direction to gain these lifelong skills. They need time to practice the social skills many of their friends seem to have learned by osmosis.

The problems that afflict ADHD youth with peers inside and outside the classroom are crucial to their sense of self and how they get along in this world. No matter what the age, knowing how to get along plays a crucial role in our sense of self.

In the next part of this chapter we will examine what medication can and cannot do to help ADHD individuals become more socially astute. As you will see, with or without medication, there are essential skills your child is likely to need to learn and use to feel good about relationships with peers.

WHAT MEDICATION CAN DO

A number of studies have been conducted to determine the effects of medication on the ADHD child's social behavior. In general, medication seems to reduce the ADHD child's aggressive, disruptive, and inappropriate behaviors. As we've noted before, on medication ADHD students look more like their peers. However, it is interesting to note that medication does not appear to improve the ADHD child's *prosocial* behaviors. In fact, very few studies have found that medication for ADHD children improves social skills.

When medication does work, it helps children focus and control impulses. It gives them a valuable edge that may improve their status in the group over time.

1. Medication Can Decrease Aggression in ADHD Youngsters.

ADHD children are "socially busy." They are drawn to and thrive on social encounters. Unfortunately, many of these encounters are aversive; that is, ADHD children may use aggressive maneuvers in order to interact with peers. For them, negative attention is better than no attention. On medication, these youth are often less discernible from their peers because they engage in fewer negative pursuits.

2. On Medication, ADHD Youngsters Can Be Less Negative and More Responsive to Parents, and Less Disruptive and Less Impulsive in the Classroom.

In interactions with adults, there is substantial improvement in cooperation. Perhaps this is not so much as to be labeled downright cooperative, but according to teacher and parent ratings, there are clearly decreases in noncompliance, defiance, and fighting.

3. On Medication, ADHD Youngsters' Status in the Group May Improve.

A study by Dr. Carol Whalen and her colleagues at the University of California reported that ADHD youth on medication had improved status in the peer group. Medication increased the number of positive descriptions, such as "fun," that peers applied to ADHD youth. In addition, because ADHD youth on medication seem to have fewer negative interactions with peers, their status within the group improves.

4. Medication *May* Help the ADHD Individual Be Receptive to Social Learning.

Anecdotal evidence from a number of clinicians who conduct social-skills classes for ADHD students indicate that medication makes a difference in the ADHD child's participation in class.

Seven-year-old Jason is the perfect example of a child who benefited from medication. When he was diagnosed at age five as ADHD, his parents wanted to try avoiding medication. Following his therapist's advice, they eagerly signed him up for a social-skills course, which met once a week, with six other ADHD kids ages six to eight years old. Each week, they worked on a specific positive social skill, for example, learning to make eye contact or accepting criticism. Jason hardly ever paid attention, and while he attended all of the classes, he simply couldn't apply the information or stay still long enough to follow the directions. The following year, after Jason was put on medication, he retook the class. Not only did he participate and learn all the skills presented, he was the star student in the class.

Medication doesn't guarantee a star student or a social butterfly. However, it may allow a child to be more fully present, able to sit still long enough to focus on the content. It may provide the opportunity for a child to become more aware of what is happening around him.

WHAT MEDICATION CANNOT DO

The effects of medication on ADHD children and youth are short-lived. They wash out with the medication. Since ADHD children generally have difficulty getting along in groups, there's a good chance that unless a child substitutes more positive social behaviors for the old ones, he will continue in his old ways both on and off medication.

1. Medication Does Not Teach Socially Acceptable Behavior.

Medication, at its best, may be thought of as a "teacher's aid." There is no clear indication that medication increases positive social interactions. Ultimately, the ADHD youngster or adult must learn positive social skills that will help him win and keep friends.

2. Medication Doesn't Help Initiate Appropriate Interactions with Peers.

Studies confirm that stimulants do not increase social interactions. Although social-skills training is an exciting trend, learning skills in a class setting doesn't automatically translate into people becoming positive social beings in the real world. On medication or not, once individuals learn specific social skills, they don't automatically put them to use. They must be prompted and reinforced to do so in daily settings.

3. Medication Does Not Help ADHD Youth or Adults Feel Happier.

A number of studies indicate that some ADHD children and adults may experience some feelings of social withdrawal as a side effect of taking stimulant medication. Sometimes youngsters report that they don't feel like interacting with their peers and may actually feel and act less social, more anxious, and sadder.

WHAT ELSE YOU CAN DO

The social problems of ADHD youth and adults are important concerns for parents and professionals. These problems contribute to the unhappiness, low self-concept, and depression many ADHD children feel. How a lack of social skills contributes to antisocial behavior later is also a question. Studies indicate that aggression is a predictor of more serious behavior problems in adulthood. Thus, helping ADHD children feel good about themselves as group members and as friends is very important. To this end, you must do more than simply give your child general advice about how to be a good friend.

KNOW YOUR OWN AND YOUR CHILD'S SOCIAL STRENGTHS AND WEAKNESSES

Each of us has strengths and weaknesses when it comes to social situations. We're most uncomfortable when we don't know how to act or what is expected of us. When we know the lay of the land, we have a comfort level that allows us to interact with others successfully.

Although some research questions whether ADHD youth are actually deficient in their knowledge of social skills, we are all aware that many times ADHD youth do not use good judgment in playing and interacting with others. They may know how to act, but they certainly don't do it. They get easily wound up in social situations or become "unglued" during transition periods. They are "socially busy," but their interactions are often aggressive and aversive.

The Social Quotient survey at the beginning of the chapter should provide you with a starting point for identifying problems. As suggested, you may gather additional insight by unobtrusively observing your child playing with others. Soliciting the opinions of other parents and teachers who have observed your child's behavior with others is also eye-opening. Use the information you collect to answer these questions.

- Which skills do you see your child using regularly?
- Where and when do most problems occur?
- Does your child know how to enter a play group?
- What does she do when others are playing nearby?
- Does he use pushing or hitting to make his presence known?
- Does she threaten to cause trouble if she doesn't get her way?
- Does he offer suggestions about what to play?
- Does she ask friends who are playing if she may join them?

REINFORCE THE USE OF SOCIAL SKILLS.

A number of studies show that the teaching of social skills in combination with behavioral reinforcement is effective in increasing appropriate social interactions and decreasing playing alone. It is important, then, to praise and reinforce your child when he displays positive social behaviors. For young children, this may take the form of specific praise. However, you will have to be more inventive in reinforcing older children and adolescents.

ARRANGE POSITIVE SOCIAL OPPORTUNITIES WITH PEERS

You can help your child interact successfully with peers by structuring positive experiences that help build interaction with peers. It's important to begin small. Limit the time your child gets together with another child, and provide structure for the time they spend together. For younger children, structure a short experience by providing an activity, a snack, and your supervision. You may alternate active play with more sedentary options. Your supervision will be important, as will your ability to head off problems and suggest solutions your child can later model.

Mrs. Bevins asked her daughter's teacher to suggest an easy playmate for Sherry. She planned for the two six-year-olds to play for two hours after school. After providing a snack, she helped them with an art activity and then supervised free play. When taking turns looked as though it might present a problem, Mrs. Bevins suggested she use her watch as a timer to give each girl an equal turn on the swing. During subsequent get-togethers, her daughter asked her mother to time herself and friends as they took turns with other toys.

PROVIDE SOCIAL-SKILLS TRAINING

ADHD youngsters are often rated as being less liked by other children. They often display behaviors that are likely to contribute to these feelings. The problem may not be lack of social skills, but lack of awareness of what is going on in a group and of the effect of their behavior on the group. Many times, ADHD individuals don't read facial cues or body language and miss other clues that cue social behaviors. In addition, sometimes their own facial expressions and body language give off inappropriate messages. Social-skills training in a group setting provides an opportunity for the child not only to learn specific skills, but to practice skills and get feedback from her peers on particular behaviors.

Social-skills training is an important, successful technique that has arisen in the past decade. Typically, social-skills training is conducted by trained counselors and therapists in order to provide children, adolescents, and their families an opportunity to learn basic social skills in a supportive environment.

Many schools have begun offering social-skills classes as part of the curriculum to enhance interpersonal relations among students. Professionals in your community may also offer courses or workshops on social skills for adults or provide such experiences during group therapy for adolescents and adults.

As our Social Quotient survey indicates, social skills can be grouped into three areas:

1. Conversational Skills
2. Building Relationships
3. Handling Emotions

Successful social-skills instruction will cover all three areas, with an emphasis on the first two, in a format that includes the elements detailed below. Most important, though, social-skills groups provide a safe place where youth and adults can learn how to look over a situation, stop and think about what to do, and then try the appropriate action.

Instruction in Specific Skills

One social-skill interchange takes a lot of work. Often it's the little things that are missed by ADHD individuals. Breaking down the skill into smaller, manageable parts makes it easier to identify what's missing, and then to teach it.

For the ADHD individual, the fact that an effective greeting includes eye contact may be what makes the skill difficult. When Jonathon's mother spoke with us about having her son join our clinic's social-skills group, she said he didn't know how to have a simple conversation with kids his own age. However, after we talked to him for only a few minutes, it was obvious that there was a more immediate problem: He didn't make eye contact. This was the first skill we taught.

There are a number of social skills that, although often taken for grant, are an important part of communication.

Expressing a Positive Attitude.

Many ADHD individuals are unaware of how their tone and demeanor affect the way others view them. In this case, seeing is believing. It's very helpful to tape-record or videotape the individual interacting with others. When the child or adult is able to see his facial expression, is able to note how looking away appears, and can view other negative aspects of his attitude, a change is often possible. The child or adult may also then be motivated to practice pleasant expressions and stances in a mirror.

Making Eye Contact.

One reason ADHD individuals miss opportunities to connect with the real world and with others is that they are focusing their attention elsewhere. Eye contact forces an individual to look at the person who is speaking, and in many cases to pick up most of what the speaker is saying. Many children will immediately get the idea if you play a game of "Radar." Have the child practice orienting his radar beam toward whoever is speaking. If the child is uncomfortable focusing on the speaker's eyes, have him look at the forehead or elsewhere on the face of the person. That's okay; those areas "work" too. Remind the child that radar acts like an invisible beam that puts you in direct contact with the individual. Practice playing Radar whenever you give directions.

Acting Interested.

One of the hardest things for many ADHD individuals is to stay interested or at least look interested. As in the game of Radar, the individual must learn to look at and listen to someone until he or she finishes speaking. Help a young child understand that an uninterested look communicates, "I don't care about you or what you're saying," and then show her how it feels to others when she appears disinterested. This can be very helpful. Have your child imagine for a moment that she just won a gold medal in the Olympics and immediately called her best friend with the news. The friend, though, was on the way out of the house and upon hearing the announcement, replied, "That's nice," and hung up. How would that feel?

Respecting Physical Boundaries.

Everyone has an invisible comfort zone. When someone invades that space, we want to back away, move, or push the person out. ADHD children, in particular, often intrude upon those boundaries by getting too close to another person, putting their hands on someone, or running up and grabbing or hitting someone. ADHD children and youth need practice in understanding what is too close, and how to stand near someone without touching. This is another time when videotaping may help the child become aware of how close he is to others and how often he may touch another person.

Reading Body Language.

ADHD individuals are like most of us: When we feel good, we stand proud; when we feel bad, we might slump. Our body language often sends out messages about how we feel about ourselves.

More important, many people become keen readers of other people's body language. We enter a room and survey the situation. Some groups of individuals place themselves in closed arrangements that make it difficult for others to join the group. Anyone has a better chance of entering a group that is open. Learning how to recognize which groups are open and which are closed is a very helpful skill. In social-skills groups, individuals can practice watching groups and using different openings to enter a group. Knowing how to "read" a group before attempting entry can be the start of more successful interactions.

Starting a Conversation.

ADHD individuals often find it difficult to approach others. They may not know how to begin a conversation. A social-skills group provides a safe place to practice a variety of conversation openers.

Dealing with Rejection.

Many ADHD youngsters are rejected by peers. Learning how to deal with rejection and to try again when rebuffed is crucial to children who have experienced disapproval before. Rehearsal with friends will prepare the child to deal with such situations.

Avoiding Disagreements.

Learning how to handle disputes is a skill most people have to learn. Mastering the art of compromise and being able to say no are also valuable tools. Within the group setting common situations in which disagreements occur are role-played and solutions discussed and tried.

Practice the Skill in a Safe Setting

A key element in the success of social-skills training is the opportunity for the participants to rehearse each skill after watching the trainer model it.

In each training session, one skill is introduced. For example, the counselor might say, "Today we are going to talk about joining a conversation." The children are then asked what are the components of the skill. After offering suggestions, the children are encouraged to discuss why specific suggestions might or might not work and what the group might do or say in return.

The leader models a specific sequence of actions for the children to take turns role-playing. These scenarios may be videotaped so that the players watch themselves and become aware of their actions.

Provide Feedback for the Individual

An interesting study of the social judgment of ADHD boys found that whether they were on medication or not, the ADHD youth could identify inappropriate social behaviors in others. In fact, boys with greater behavior problems themselves were the best judges of the behavior of others.

However, recognizing what other people are doing right and wrong and giving appropriate feedback are two different things. Again, the therapist plays a valuable role in modeling and teaching group participants to give both positive and constructive feedback to their peers.

Often, reviewing the videotape is one of the most useful elements of social-skills training. Seeing yourself in action is truly an experience worth a thousand lectures. Brad was a twelve-year-old who participated in one of our first social-skills groups. A bright, energetic, and impulsive youngster, he was always ready to contribute to the classes, but had difficulty accepting instruction. Brad had been told repeatedly by his group that he didn't look anyone in the face when he was talking. He didn't believe it until he watched himself on camera. He really thought he had been practicing making eye contact, but it was obvious that after a second or two he began looking elsewhere. When he practiced the skill in the group, he still found it very difficult to look anyone in the eye. He was able, though, to look "in the area" of someone's face.

Prompt Use of the Skill

It is very important to incorporate into social-skills training the ability to transfer the newly learned skills to natural settings. Often students in social-skills groups are given specific assignments after sessions to prompt them to use their new skills. In some groups, participants are encouraged to bring a good friend to particular sessions so that they will have a peer to practice with later. Successful and unsuccessful attempts in a natural setting can then be discussed with the rest of the group.

Reinforce Appropriate Use of Skills

Promoting the use of new social skills can also be heightened through the use of praise and reinforcement. Children should be praised for all attempts to use the skills they are learning. A "good behavior diary," in which the parent records each attempt the child makes to use a new social skill, can be a positive way to praise and prompt appropriate behavior. In addition, rewards can be very effective tools to encourage children to use the skills in new settings.

A FINAL WORD ON SOCIAL SKILLS

Learning how to live, work, and play with others is crucial to a happy life. Research indicates that children without friends who are isolated from their peers are at risk for continuing problems with peers, poor academic achievement, and poor adjustment to school. At the very least, children who are socially isolated have no opportunity to learn how to function and live as a member of a group.

Social-skills training in coordination with behavior management and reinforcement can be a valuable way for children and adolescents to learn the skills they have not adopted otherwise. Impulsive children need a safe place where they can wait, observe, and rehearse the skill they need. Children who are "socially busy" in a negative way need to learn how to redirect their social efforts in a manner that brings about the friendships they desire. Whether ADHD youngsters are on medication or not, social-skills training is an important part of their reeducation.

8

RECHANNELING THE ADHD MIND

Learning Self-Control

"Why don't you stop and think before you do things?"
"Please! Learn to control yourself!"

If you have an ADHD youngster or are an ADHD adult, you have probably said and/or heard statements like these too many times to count. Although fidgetiness and overactivity may annoy others more, the characteristic that plagues individuals with ADHD the most is their inability to control their thoughts, their actions, and sometimes their emotions. It is this impulsiveness to speak, act, and feel that gets them off track, disrupts their routines, and plays havoc with their daily lives.

As an adult with ADHD, you may have developed great control in some areas, but may still feel out of control in others. The fact that you must put food on the table may keep you going to work each day, but you may be quick to react when your boss or coworker questions your judgment or actions. You may adhere to a schedule at the office, but your workshop may be a mess. Or your timetable for paying bills might be so erratic that some bills have been paid twice and others are overdue.

Imposing structure on the daily activities of ADHD children is an effective way to help them control their behavior. Yet even as parents and teachers work diligently to do that, they wish and pray that the children will develop "self-control."

So how do you go about developing self-control in your child or yourself? To answer these questions we must first look at why those with ADHD often have trouble controlling their thoughts and impulses.

WHY DO PEOPLE WITH ADHD
HAVE TROUBLE WITH SELF-CONTROL?

Because ADHD is not a simple problem, there is not a single, simple answer to this question. Rather, there are several factors that play a part in the self-control issue for ADHD people.

1. ADHD Individuals Find It Difficult to Ignore External Distractions.

One of the first things you notice about individuals with ADHD is how easily they get distracted by things around them. Watch an ADHD student in the classroom. He's the first to look up when a classmate clears his throat. Observe an ADHD adult working at her desk. A bird flies past the window, and she automatically tracks it instead of the line of numbers she is adding for a report. Admonitions to ignore distractions and "keep your eye on the paper" or "keep your mind on your work" are useless.

2. ADHD Individuals Have Trouble Controlling Their Own Thoughts.

Dr. Russell Barkley emphasizes that the core feature of ADHD is the inability to control the impulses that disrupt attention. Given this, then the question of which came first—short attention or distractibility—is quite clear. ADHD is not a problem of short attention; it is a problem of control. The inability to control one's thoughts, actions, or movements disrupts attention.

Unfortunately, youth and adults with ADHD are not simply distracted by things in the environment. They also have trouble controlling the impulses that lead from one thought to the next. One of the young men we worked with describes his mind as a television set with a broken remote control. Not only does it continually change channels, he doesn't know how to turn off the set.

Many ADHD youths identify with this picture. Like a television viewer continually flipping from one station to another, channel surfing from idea to idea, their concentration is continually interrupted by random thoughts, feelings, and physical sensations.

Ten-year-old Jeremie recounted in one of our sessions how his mind worked. His description is a classic: "I was sitting in math class before lunch and noticed that I was hungry. Then I started thinking about what we might be having for lunch in the cafeteria and what I really wanted to eat—my favorite dinner is one my Grandma makes: meatballs and brown rice. Somehow, I then started thinking about the last family reunion and how my cousin and I found a frog. Suddenly, the teacher called my name and asked me for my answer to the math question."

Of course, all Jeremie could do at that moment was look at his teacher with a blank stare, since he had no idea what question she had asked. Jeremie's thoughts were like dominoes. Once the pattern began, one thought toppled into the next until something stopped the flow.

No wonder people with ADHD often have trouble staying focused even when they are not distracted by external stimuli. If you can't control the direction or speed of your thoughts, you are also likely to have trouble controlling your actions in many situations.

3. ADHD Individuals Can Get Overfocused.

Sometimes people with ADHD have the opposite problem: They become overfocused. Consider the child who is locked into a video game or who is glued to the television screen. His concentration converges on that one activity to such a degree he doesn't hear his name called or anything else that is occurring around him. It is not unusual to hear a parent describe his ADHD child by saying, "When he's hooked into something, a freight train could come through the room and he wouldn't hear it."

You might think such application to one activity is "selective attention" on your child's part, especially when you are calling him to a chore. In fact, however, this is not always a matter of the ADHD youngster's electing not to hear a parent but is rather a matter of being driven to continue the action.

Adults, too, can become overfocused. A young stockbroker who had recently been diagnosed ADHD said he often found himself becoming so focused on tracking the activity of certain stocks, he forgot to make the client calls he had scheduled.

Sometimes the problem is not simply one of becoming overfocused but rather one of focusing on the wrong details. Terrell, a bright eleventh-grader, indicated one reason he wanted to try medication again was that he never focused on the right things: "I'm so busy trying to hear my teacher and trying to keep myself concentrating on what she's saying that I don't notice important messages on the board. I missed a note last week about a test."

Being able to control your attention—determining what you pay attention to, when you pay attention, and for how long—is as crucial to success as having a long attention span.

4. Rewards Are Not as Strong a Motivator for
ADHD Individuals as They Are for Their Peers.

As we mentioned in Chapter 4, there is a growing body of research that indicates that people who suffer from ADHD do not react as others do to the same consequences. Positive consequences don't appear to be as strong a motivator as they are for other children.

Some researchers have theorized that the threshold for reinforcement in the brain of people with ADHD is set too high. In order for a reward to influence behavior it must be stronger and more immediate than those typically used. When rewards are delayed or given less frequently, they seem to lose their effectiveness more quickly.

What this means is that although ADHD youth may want to earn a good grade or receive their weekly allowance, they are often unable to control their behavior to achieve those ends. You may have discovered this yourself. Do you find yourself continually raising the ante or offering your child larger and larger rewards to get him to behave? Or you may have given up on rewards, concluding that they simply don't work for your child.

Being the parent of an ADHD child does change a parent's behavior. Several researchers who studied the behavior of mothers of ADHD children found them to be more directive and negative with their ADHD children than they were with non-ADHD children. These findings suggest that somewhere deep down these mothers gave up on praise and positive reinforcement to control their children.

ADHD adults who are laboring for much larger rewards often have trouble motivating themselves to work for delayed gratification. Even people who are vastly successful in one area may have great difficulty harnessing their attention in other areas. Others who are enthusiastic at the beginning of a job are likely to become bored and turned off quickly, regardless of the salary or other inducements.

5. Negative Consequences Do Not Have the Same Impact on Behavior.

Not only are positive consequences less effective with ADHD youngsters and adults, potential negative consequences also seem to have less impact on behavior. For example, the fear of getting a bad grade is often not enough to motivate the ADHD student to study, as much as it might his classmates. Similarly, an ADHD adult may not be sufficiently motivated to act by the negative consequences of missing a deadline at work.

Researchers have suggested that understimulation in those centers of the brain that control inhibition may cause people with ADHD to adapt more quickly to negative consequences. In other words, they tend to underreact to the possible negative impact of an action so that they react only at the last minute and only to very dire consequences.

This decreased sensitivity to both positive and negative consequences often causes people with ADHD to seem (and feel) as if they are not in control of themselves or their lives.

6. ADHD Individuals Have Difficulty Adhering to Rules.

The old saying, "Rules are made to be broken," seems to have been created by youngsters with ADHD. Although many youngsters and adults break rules occasionally, ADHD youth have continual problems adhering to rules at home, at school, and elsewhere.

It is proposed by a number of researchers that at its heart, ADHD is a deficit in rule-governed behavior. A rule is a customary action or a standard of behavior that relates to what is commonly good for everyone. A rule may be written, like the speed limit on highways, or understood (for example, brushing your teeth after you eat).

Rules typically have defined or implied consequences, either positive or negative. A positive rule specifies an action that must be done, as well as its reward, which may be stated or implied. Its counterpart is the negative consequence for not complying with the rule. "Brush your teeth after meals and you will get fewer cavities" is an example of a positive rule. "Break the speed limit and you will get a speeding ticket" illustrates a negative rule.

Although some ADHD youngsters may be so oppositional that they break rules on purpose, most have trouble following rules for other reasons. They may not pay attention to the rule, so that they simply don't notice the sign that says KEEP OFF THE GRASS. Similarly, it's not uncommon for ADHD students to forget to read the directions for an assignment. Other times, they may have noted the rule but forgotten when to follow it or what they were supposed to do. In these cases, out of sight is indeed out of mind, for the student is already on to other things.

Finally, ADHD youth are sometimes so impulsive that even though they are aware of a rule, they act without thinking before they realize they are breaking the rule. For example, your child may know the rule about looking both ways before crossing the street, but when his favorite ball rolls into the street, he impulsively runs after it without a thought to the rule. Obviously, the failure to follow rules can have disastrous consequences.

7. ADHD Individuals Don't Learn From Corrections.

Few people like being reminded to do something or having their behavior corrected. Parents and teachers often find themselves constantly reminding and directing ADHD youngsters. In some cases, adults feel as though supervising these youths is a full-time job. On the other side of the coin, children and especially teenagers who suffer from ADHD hate being reminded, corrected, and otherwise controlled continually. Similarly, adults with ADHD often resent the frequent prompting or nagging by spouses and others. In fact, everyone—ADHD youth and adults, their friends and relatives—wishes that things could be different. As we've stated, however, rarely is there evidence that the ADHD individual outgrows the pattern.

WHAT MEDICATION CAN DO

Medication can improve certain aspects of functioning that may lead to improvements in control.

1. Medication Can Decrease Impulsivity.

Individuals who respond to medication often show a decrease in impulsiveness. Their improvement is most noticeable in terms of overt behavior, so that children do not interrupt as often or blurt out answers to questions in class. On written work, students and adults may show a decrease in the number of careless errors they make, and they may be less frustrated so that they are less quick to anger when they meet a difficult task. In this way, on medication ADHD individuals stay on a task longer without switching activities. In social situations, individuals appear to have greater control so that they act less aggressively.

2. Medication May Lower the Threshold for Reinforcement.

There is some evidence that medication may increase responsiveness to reinforcement. It's speculated this may be due to a lowering of the threshold for reinforcement, or it simply may be because the person is paying greater attention to the contingencies that lead to reinforcement. Whatever the cause, it appears that on medication some individuals, children and older individuals alike, can delay gratification for longer periods of time so that they continue working to earn the reinforcement whether the reinforcement is delayed or intermittent.

3. Medication May Improve Responsiveness to Punishment.

As is the case with reinforcement, individuals on medication are more responsive to negative consequences such as punishment. It's speculated that medication improves the ability of the brain to control motor inhibition so that children can inhibit responses that would lead to punishment, or helps the child become more aware of the consequences of behavior that leads to punishment. In either case, experiencing punishment or thinking about future negative consequences may then lead to improvement in control.

4. Medication May Improve Compliance to Rules.

ADHD youth who respond to medication follow the rules more often. Consequently, they get into less trouble. Again, this may be caused by a decrease in impulsiveness or better attention to directions. Or it may be due to greater awareness of both the positive and negative consequences of their behavior.

WHAT MEDICATION CANNOT DO

Many people categorize ADHD individuals, especially those who are not hyperactive, as "absentminded professor" types who always have lots of ideas about what to do and how to do it. Such creative thinkers are very valuable. However, "divergent" thinking may result in nothing more than spinning one's wheels unless the individual learns to translate those thoughts into productive problem solving. Unfortunately, this part doesn't come naturally to most people with ADHD, and medication does not teach them what to focus on and when to lock and unlock their selective attention.

1. Medication Does Not Teach Reflective Thinking.

Even if medication decreases overt impulsive behavior, it does not teach internal reflective thinking. Some situations require what is known as "convergent" thinking, in which all effort is directed toward one solution for quick decision making. People with ADHD are sometimes very good at making quick decisions. For example, you hear on the radio that there are limited tickets available for your favorite group's upcoming concert. You make an instant decision to drop what you are doing and hurry to the box office. As a result of your quick decision and concentrated effort, you are able to purchase front-row seats. Onlookers and relatives may call your behavior "impulsive," but you now hold the best tickets in town.

In other situations such quick action can lead to less impressive results or to problems. An older teenager and his parents came to see us after the young man bought a used car he "fell in love with." True, he paid for it with money he had earned, but he failed to have anyone check out the car for mechanical problems; he hadn't even considered other cars. Without discussing this major purchase with anyone, he gave an acquaintance $750 and drove a lemon home. Everyone would probably agree that a little less single-mindedness and a little more reflection, including some divergent thinking about the "what ifs," would have been prudent in this situation. Medication may slow down impulsive behavior, but it does not teach reflective thinking or problem solving.

2. Medication Does Not Teach You How to Control Where to Focus Attention.

Knowing what to pay attention to is just as important as paying attention. On medication, ADHD individuals may concentrate and sustain their attention longer, but they do not automatically know what to focus their attention on or when and how to switch their attention. This is the main reason why so many ADHD students, even on medication, continue to have problems with social situations or transition periods. Complicating most situations is the fact that, although they may listen intently and better observe what is going on, many ADHD youths just don't recognize the clues body language offers and the changes in tone of voice that others quickly note. Medication cannot teach these individuals the elements of a situation that require their attention. (See Chapter 7.)

3. Medication Does Not Increase the Child's Motivation to Control Behavior.

Although medication may improve sensitivity to both positive and negative consequences, it doesn't supply the will to conform. As many parents and teachers of ADHD youngsters will attest, medication does not improve overall motivation or "attitude." The same is true of ADHD adults. Even on medication, many people with ADHD have trouble motivating themselves to start projects and complete tasks. Unfortunately, there is no evidence that medication teaches ADHD individuals how to set attainable goals and how to reach them.

4. Medication Does Not Teach ADHD Individuals How to Control Anger.
Many youngsters and adults with ADHD have trouble handling frustration and anger. This is of particular concern, since trouble controlling
anger and controlling aggression are two aspects of ADHD that may be
predictors of future problems. In this case, medication may decrease the
individual's frustration and improve impulse control, but it will not teach
him how to deal with anger or other feelings.

WHAT ELSE YOU CAN DO

The retroactive studies by Weiss and Hechtman conducted at Montreal
Children's Hospital of ADHD children grown up often found that ADHD
adults whose only form of treatment during childhood was medication
remained impulsive. Their impulsiveness as they aged, however, took
more ominous forms. They had more children out of wedlock, had more
automobile accidents, changed jobs more often, and lived in more homes
over the years. One might convincingly argue that these behaviors reflect
a certain amount of impulsiveness on their part.

For years, clinicians and researchers have been searching for ways to
help ADHD youth with the aspects of this disorder that are often not
improved even when medication works on the "core symptoms." A major focus of the inquiry remains improving self-control.

In the early 1970s, there was a great deal of excitement generated by
the work of Dr. Donald Meichenbaum. In 1971, Drs. Meichenbaum and
Goodman published an article in the *Journal of Abnormal Psychology* entitled "Training Impulsive Children to Talk to Themselves: A Means of
Developing Self-Control." In this study and those that followed, numerous researchers tried using what is labeled as *cognitive-behavioral therapy*
to teach self-control.

Cognitive-behavioral therapy focused on first changing what a person thinks and feels, which in turn would then lead to changes in overt
behavior. These are commonly referred to as *stop, look,* and *listen* techniques. When this approach is used with ADHD youngsters, the child
is first taught a series of steps to help him stop, think, and problem-
solve before responding. In the original studies conducted by Dr.
Meichenbaum and others, students who learned cognitive behavioral
techniques showed improvement in specific scores on tests that require
reflective thinking.

Later studies of cognitive-behavioral interventions looked at actual classroom behaviors. A 1976 study by Drs. Bornstein and Quevillon targeted actual on-task behavior in preschoolers. After only two hours of cognitive-behavioral training, these students' on-task behavior improved. Even more remarkably, these improvements lasted for months.

As you might imagine, many clinicians were excited by these results and were anxious to apply the findings of cognitive-behavioral therapy. After all, people have been telling ADHD children for years to "stop and think before acting." Unfortunately, other researchers who have tried to replicate the promising results of the early cognitive-therapy studies with other ADHD youngsters have not found similar real or lasting effects. Most positive effects of cognitive-behavior therapy, without medication, have been noted in laboratory studies, and instances in which improvement was noted still did not produce as great an improvement as medication alone. In general, self-instructional training in which the child is taught to "stop, look, and listen" has not been shown to generalize from laboratory procedures to classroom settings or elsewhere unless other behavioral techniques are included.

However, that is not to say that cognitive-behavioral interventions have no value in the treatment of ADHD. In their 1985 book *Cognitive-Behavioral Therapy for Impulsive Children*, Drs. Philip Kendall and Lauren Braswell reviewed the results of many studies of the cognitive mediation of behavior. They concluded that cognitive strategies, when accompanied by behavioral contingencies, could be effective in reducing impulsiveness.

A variety of techniques are included under the heading of cognitive-behavioral interventions. These include behavioral self-control techniques such as self-monitoring and self-reinforcement.

INTRODUCE SELF-MONITORING

One step toward self-control is self-monitoring. The research clearly indicates that children can be taught to observe and record their own behavior. An ADHD child can be taught to monitor her behavior at particular times and to note whether she is on-task or not. In such situations, some sort of auditory or visual stimulus such as a beep or hand signal is usually given, and the child records whether she is on-task at that moment.

The ripple effects of self-monitoring look quite promising. Self-monitoring combined with reinforcement has been shown to be effective in improving attention. In a study conducted by Drs. Neilans and Israel in 1981, the researchers found that having a child mark whether or not he was on-task at particular moments in time decreased disruptive behavior by one third.

At times the child not only monitors his own behavior, but reinforces himself when his performance indicates. Self-reinforcement then involves an additional level of evaluation. Self-management and self-reinforcement have been shown to be effective adjuncts in classrooms where the teacher is unable to monitor or reinforce a student's behavior.

Although more research is needed in this area, it is reasonable to hypothesize that cognitive-behavioral therapy would be a significant element of treatment for adults with ADHD. A number of clinicians have suggested that cognitive strategies work better with older and more verbal people. Furthermore, if ADHD is viewed as a problem of motivation, then it would appear that cognitive-behavioral psychotherapy might be an important element of treatment for adults with ADHD. Understanding and dealing with one's thoughts and emotions are essential to feeling liked and being in better control.

LEARN THE STEPS TO PROBLEM SOLVING

Problem solving is an essential skill for individuals of all ages. You can enhance your youngster's and your own ability to think reflectively by learning specific steps in the problem-solving process. By definition, if you use this process, you cannot be impulsive.

On the basis of the work of cognitive behaviorists, the steps to the problem-solving process might include the following elements.

1. Define the Problem.

Stop and ask yourself, "What is the problem I need to solve?" For example, you have to complete a summer reading assignment. You ask yourself, "Exactly what is it I must do to complete my reading assignment?" The answer might be, "Read five books and write a one-page report on each."

2. List the Possible Solutions.

This is the time when it is important to engage in divergent thinking. In this case, you would list all of the possible approaches to solving the problem. You might ask yourself, "What are all of the ways that I could meet my summer reading requirement?" Your list might include:

- Pick the first five books on the list.
- Pick five novels on the list.
- Pick five biographies on the list.
- Pick a mixture of books.
- Ask the teacher if I could read certain books not on the list.

3. Focus Attention on the Problem.

While thinking of possible solutions to the problem, you deliberately inhibit other thoughts and ignore external distractions that could interrupt your concentration. You might say to yourself, "I must continue working on this problem until I decide which books I will read."

4. Choose One Solution.

Now is the time for convergent thinking in order to bring about a decision. You might consider the possibilities and conclude, "I need to choose one approach before I lose my concentration. I will read five novels."

5. Try Your Solution.

No amount of thinking about creative problem solving is of any value unless you carry the plan into action. This is the step at which many people with ADHD get caught. For them, the solution often means that the behavior must be prompted. For example, you might remind yourself: "I will now open up this book and read the foreword."

6. Self-Reinforce or Self-Correct.

If your solution was a good one, at least give yourself a pat on the back. Better yet, reward yourself by doing something you would enjoy. Begin by saying, "I did a good job and chose the right books to read." If you made a mistake, make a coping statement such as, "I made a mistake. This looked like a good book, but I will get through it and try another one next time." If you need to change your solution, do so now. "I will read a biography next."

MODEL ON OTHERS WHO HAVE
GOOD SELF-CONTROL STRATEGIES

Many of the self-control programs have a built-in modeling component in which children do and say to themselves what they see a "coach" doing. You can serve as your child's coach by showing him how you use the problem-solving steps as you encounter various situations.

One way to begin is to contrive situations in which you demonstrate problem-solving skills that your child could use. Many ADHD children are easily frustrated. To increase problem solving in such situations, use a puzzle or game as an opportunity to teach problem solving. For example, if you are playing checkers, you can say out loud, "Wait a minute. I have got to look at all my possible moves. Oh, if I move there he will jump me! Here is a better move!" Over time, model problem-solving steps in every-day situations.

Adults can also learn from models. If you are comfortable with the situation, you may find that a relative or good friend is willing to serve as a model for you, even if he or she doesn't overtly use all of the same steps to solve problems. Observe how the individual goes about certain tasks. Ask questions about how he approaches the task and why he chose a particular strategy. Ask the individual to explain to you what other possibilities he considered and discarded. You may find the person is also comfortable talking about the process he goes through when a solution does not work. Most important, be sure to ask how he keeps his focus on solving the problem.

Copy and complete the Steps to Problem Solving form in Table 8.1 to practice reflective-thinking skills.

Table 8.1

Steps to Problem Solving

1. What is the problem?

_____

_____

2. What are all the possible solutions I can think of?

_____

_____

_____

_____

3. How can I focus on this problem until it is resolved?

_____

_____

4. What is my chosen solution?

_____

_____

5. How will I go about trying the solution?

_____

_____

_____

6. How will I reinforce myself or self-correct?

_____

_____

_____

VERBALIZE YOUR INTENTIONS

Whether you are an adult or a child, when you are at the early part of the learning cycle, it is very important to make each step conspicuous. As you go about problem solving, verbalize each step you are taking. This is important because it not only forces you to stick to the plan, but combats impulsiveness. Utter each step:

1. Identify the problem.
2. Generate possible solutions.
3. Explain how you are keeping your mind on solving the problem.
4. Isolate the solution you have decided to try first.
5. Indicate how you are going to start.
6. Determine what you are going to say to yourself if the solution does or doesn't work.

If you are acting as your child's coach, verbalize the steps a few times yourself, then have the youngster do the same. Like any good coach, praise your youngster as she does each step, and prompt her if she gets off track. If you find your child really gets stuck, model the skill again.

As an adult, you may find it more comfortable to rehearse the problem-solving techniques in private before committing yourself publicly. As you become confident of the process, you may find that whispering or subvocalizing the steps is also successful. People overhearing your mutterings may label you slightly eccentric at most.

INTERNALIZE SELF-TALK

Moving from verbalization to subvocalization is the interim step as you or your child learns to simply "think" about what it is that must be done. Begin by practicing making statements to yourself that help you stay on-task. You might find it productive to write standard questions on index cards that can be used to prompt thoughtful problem solving. For example, if you have to read some material, you might ask yourself or have your child estimate how many pages you read without looking up or daydreaming. Statements such as, "Keep your eyes on the paper," "Ignore those people walking by," and "I will think about what else I need to do later," may prompt on-task behavior.

TEACH CHILDREN AND ADULTS TO MONITOR THEIR OWN ATTENDING

Some research has shown that youngsters can improve their self-control and on-task behavior by self-monitoring. In our book, *Is Your Child*

Hyperactive? Inattentive? Impulsive? Distractible?, we described several techniques that have been effective in lengthening children's attention span for a task. In one technique, based on cognitive-behavioral techniques of self-monitoring, the parent sets a timer for varying periods of time as a child works on a homework task. If the child is on-task at the moment the timer rings, he is awarded a point. Next, have the child set the timer for himself. When the bell rings, have the child determine whether he is on-task. If you agree with his evaluation, award the child a point. After a number of such agreements you can begin to remove yourself from the monitoring by checking less often.

Combining self-monitoring with token reinforcement or response cost (see Chapter 4) has been shown to be an effective way to teach self-evaluation. Dr. Harvey Parker, Co-Founder and Past Executive Director of Ch.A.D.D., a national support group for children and adults with ADHD, has produced an audiotape that has beeping tones at varying intervals along with self-monitoring forms. Information about this and other materials is presented at the end of this book in the Resources section.

Table 8.2 is an example of a Self-Monitoring-Record. You may make an audiotape for your child with a beeper or bell sounding at random intervals ranging from thirty seconds to five minutes.

USE SELF-REINFORCEMENT

There are many appealing elements of cognitive-behavioral training. Everyone wants children to feel better about their own behavior. Learning to self-reward after a job well done is one step toward this goal.

Several studies have shown that children can be taught to accurately rate their own behavior. Begin by having a child evaluate his own behavior at various steps during the problem-solving process. Role-play statements that can be made to reinforce appropriate behavior, such as, "I did a good job of defining the problem," "I read three pages as I said I would." Compare the child's assessment with your own to determine the child's accuracy, and praise your child for accuracy.

Table 8.2

Self-Monitoring Record

Directions:	TIMED INTERVAL	ON-TASK	OFF-TASK
1. Use a prerecorded audiotape or set a timer for varying intervals ranging from thirty seconds to five minutes.	1	*	
	2	*	
	3		*
	4	*	
	5		*
	6	*	
2. As the child does an assignment, have him indicate whether he is on-task at the moment the bell rings. Verify your child's assessment until you are assured of his accuracy.	7		*
	8		*
	9		*
	10	*	
	TOTAL	**5/10**	**5/10** **50% ON-TASK**

3. Record the number of times the child is on-task and divide it by the number of intervals to determine the on-task percentage. An example is provided.	TIMED INTERVAL	ON-TASK	OFF-TASK
	1		
	2		
	3		
	4		
	5		
	6		
	7		
	8		
	9		
	10		
	TOTAL/PERCENT		

A FINAL WORD ABOUT SELF-CONTROL TRAINING

Impulsiveness is an ongoing concern of parents and individuals with ADHD. Many treatment strategies have been reported in the literature, and certainly every parent, teacher, clinician, and researcher desires to find ways to help ADHD youth and adults develop self-control. Unfortunately, the results of most of the research efforts are not yet clear. Often treatments such as cognitive-behavioral interventions work to teach children to mediate their behavior through self-instruction appear to yield positive results in the lab, but these results don't hold up for the long run or in real-life settings.

Cognitive-behavioral intervention strategies that teach ADHD youth to "stop, think, listen" and "problem-solve" are very appealing because they address the core problem of ADHD. While medication alone is not an effective solution, medication and behavior-management strategies—including reinforcement and response cost coupled with self-instruction, self-monitoring, and self-reinforcement—do have promise in teaching self-control.

9

ROUTINES MEDICATION DOESN'T TEACH

Building Organization Skills for Life

W hen you review the diagnostic criteria for ADHD in *DSM-IV*, it is obvious that disorganization is a key element of the disorder. The criteria include:

- Often has difficulty organizing thoughts and activities.
- Often has difficulty organizing tasks and activities.
- Often loses things for organizing tasks or activities.
- Often is forgetful in daily activity.

Even when medication has a positive effect on other aspects of ADHD, these are some of the characteristics that seem to be least improved by medication.

Eleven-year-old LISA *is a walking mass of assorted papers, pens, incomplete homework assignments, should-have-been-discarded candy wrappers, and yet-to-be-found sweaters, jackets, and misplaced books. Frequently told she's an accident waiting to happen, she'll do her homework, only to discover the next day she did the wrong assignment or omitted problems. Yet her standard reply to the question, "Do you have homework to do?" is "I've done it all." She really believes that's true.*

Medication helped Lisa be more attentive and less distractible so that she was able to correctly record the assigned homework in her assignment book more often, and to complete her classwork more punctually. She still *found herself doing book reports and completing projects at the last minute. In other words, Ritalin didn't automatically teach*

Lisa how to break down a task and get everything to the right place at the right time. Ritalin doesn't teach organizational skills.

If you are a parent or spouse of someone with ADHD, most mornings you probably feel like a traffic cop looking in every direction to prevent accidents. You know that unless you conscientiously scrutinize the situation, someone is bound to leave the house without his or her books, tote, briefcase, glasses, or wallet, or any number of other essentials.

ADHD folks are notorious for leaving, losing, or misplacing things. As one parent of an eight-year-old told us, "Brad can't keep up with anything. Every evening and every morning is a marathon ordeal." Brad, in his understated manner, dryly acknowledged, "It's really hard for me to keep up with everything."

Some people seem to be born organized. Others naturally recognize the advantage routines have for them and struggle to put good habits in place. Sometimes ADHD youth, and adults, seem incapable of adopting such habits.

Twelve-year-old **ADRIENNE** *had the assignment book, the book bag, and a time and a place to do homework. Her parents even hired a tutor who specialized in study skills to help her get organized. Her homework record improved as long as both parents took turns watching her like a hawk. Each evening one or the other cross-checked each task with the assignment book, then made sure the sheet was in the proper notebook in the book bag, and that the book bag was by the bedroom door before bedtime. When they stopped checking, Adrienne reverted to old habits. Within a week after the cross-checking stopped, papers were placed haphazardly in the book bag, and sometimes assignments were forgotten. Adrienne didn't habituate the new routines. She acknowledged she needed to, but even her teachers' telling her she could probably raise most of her subject grades by an entire letter if she'd only get organized didn't cause her to change.*

GETTING A HANDLE ON DISORGANIZATION

Adrienne and many other ADHD individuals must have a clear motivation to overcome chronic disorganization. The unfortunate truth is that until negative consequences register strongly enough, disorganization typically thrives. One ADHD father, who struggled to untangle his disorganized habits for years, admitted that one particular disaster changed his ways. He told us the final straw came for him when he missed the deadline on a financial deal because the letter was buried in hundreds of papers on his desk. That cost him several thousand dollars.

Ryan found the motivation to get his act together. A junior in high school, he has severe attention deficit disorder without hyperactivity. Ritalin helps him manage his distractibility, but he has always been disorganized. He does most papers at the last minute and always finds himself cramming for exams.

Sometimes the stress of his situation shows itself in what might be called temper tantrums. His anger would flare with little provocation but did nothing to help him meet deadlines, find papers, or get ready on time.

Ryan went through something of a miracle change his last year in high school. He wanted to be an actor. He was quite talented and had been in numerous local productions, but his grades were not good enough to get into the acting school of his choice. With assistance from his teachers, he identified a series of rules or "must do's" for each day. Ryan made a conscious decision to stick to his plan. For example, each day he made a list of what he had to accomplish that day. He kept materials and books in one place at home and in school. Although it may seem amazing to parents of other ADHD adolescents, this young man got into acting school and accomplished his goal, not because of the medication, but because of a well-balanced approach to his disorganization.

Unfortunately, many adults, both ADHD and those without an excuse, simply adapt to the inconvenience of disorganization. They've retraced their steps and redone things for so long, it's a way of living. They simply deal with the clutter, confusion, and mess.

Disorganization uses up time and energy. Keeping up with books, bags, briefcases, and necessities is a constant strain on someone with ADHD. Imagine if you saw each attempt to complete a task, put a piece of paper in its proper place, or find an object as an isolated occurrence, unrelated, without rhyme or reason. For many with ADHD, the day is a series of such isolated occurrences. And, like other unrelated tasks, they are forgotten. So homework may be done, but it's left on the desk; a coat may be taken to school only to be left there when the afternoon warms up.

Organization means "planning and execution of an action in a systematic way over time." As you know, this skill is in complete opposition to most ADHD individuals' intrinsic nature and natural abilities. Of course, that doesn't let everyone else who is disorganized off the hook. Lots of people who are not ADHD are disorganized. Getting organized is hard for most people. The difference is that *getting organized is crucial to the success of the ADHD youth or adult.* Other people may be able to bluff it. ADHD adults and children can't fake this one.

Do you remember playing with building blocks or watching a toddler working to build a tower? You can erect a tower only so tall with single blocks; it gets wobbly fairly quickly. Add an infrastructure and the tower can become a much larger and taller building of blocks.

Children and adults with ADHD need that structure. They have difficulty regulating their own behavior over time to meet future goals. Breaking down a task into a sequence of jobs, starting at point *A* and getting to point *C,* anticipating the consequences of what might result from future actions, and learning from past results do not come naturally to them. Unfortunately, recognizing the need to get organized, and adhering to the routines that keep one organized, simply isn't automatic either.

Medication may play a role in helping your child or yourself get organized. But it still takes will as well as hard work to build the routines that are needed to keep you or your child organized.

In this chapter, we'll present a system and many tips that have helped both young and older ADHD individuals. Our hope is to encourage you to put into place a structure that will help make organization obtainable.

WHAT MEDICATION CAN DO

Although disorganization is a common outcome of ADHD, very little research has been done in this area. Several studies that have been done relate to the area called "executive functioning." Often ADHD individuals seem to have the skills and knowledge about how to organize, but don't apply the strategies when performing tasks. In approaching most tasks, they are often impulsive and inefficient. They also have difficulty articulating to others how they will go about completing a job, which meshes with their difficulty in developing and following rules.

In order to explain to someone else your strategy for completing a task, you must have developed procedures or "rules" to follow. In order to develop a plan to complete any project, you must break down the task into a series of individual actions that lead to the goal. Then, to fulfill the goal, you must follow the predetermined steps. The lack of these skills is a key problem for ADHD children.

It is probably clear to you from your own experience (and the research backs you up) that the major strategies that discriminate ADHD students from their peers include inability to work in an organized manner over time to solve a problem. What is so frustrating is that it is not the ADHD child's or adult's inability to reach the right answer that is in question. They can figure out what *B* is; they just can't always get there from *A* when they need to.

You've probably heard it a thousand times about your child, or it may echo in your mind from your own youth: "It's not that he's not bright. He simply doesn't apply himself." ADHD children have difficulty following through on an assignment, completing tasks in the requested format, working in a timely fashion, or knowing how to take notes and study. One preteen got the right answer most of the time on most of the problems of his math tests. However, he also lost half the points for each problem because he didn't remember to show his work, did not label the answer, or completed only one part of the question.

Although neither Ritalin nor any other medication will create a system for getting organized or teach a child study skills, medication can help a child or adult be more receptive to creating, learning, and maintaining an organizational scheme.

1. Medication May Increase the Effective Use of Time.

On medication, the ADHD individual uses time more efficiently, and so students complete more work.

2. On Medication, Handwriting Is Often Improved.

Keep a collection of your child's school papers completed while he is on and off medication. Compare your child's or your own handwriting on and off medication. Sometimes the comparison is dramatic. On medication, letters are formed more intentionally and spacing is more appropriate. The size and shape of letters and numbers are more uniform.

From dittos in elementary school to lecture notes in college, students of all ages are required to write a lot in most classrooms. The simple fact that writing is easier and the result more legible helps the student organize a page, align numerals, and reread notes. The same can be true for ADHD adults.

3. On Medication, ADHD Individuals Are Less Distractible and Less Impulsive.

One of the impediments to organization is interruption and disruption. It is difficult to plan ahead or to execute a task in a consecutive manner if you are constantly interrupted by thoughts and stimuli around you. On medication, many children and adults report they are able to stay with a task, read a complete page, or finish an assignment. They are less likely to sabotage their own efforts.

Medication may also settle down the impulsive behavior that accompanies ADHD, and may give a child or adult an edge for maintaining learned organizational skills.

4. Medication May Decrease Emotional Reactivity.

Many ADHD children display wide mood swings and have little tolerance for frustration or suggestions to remedy a situation. On medication, emotions may be "smoothed out," so youngsters and older individuals with ADHD are more receptive to suggestions that help them structure their time and activities.

WHAT MEDICATION CANNOT DO

Nothing—including medication—teaches an individual how to get organized. It won't teach you where to put your keys so you won't have to search for them when it's time to leave. It won't make your child get up on time or teach her to lay out her clothes and prepare her book bag the night before so she can be ready on time for school. In other words, it won't create the valuable routines that will help you avoid the problems that make you late and add to your procrastination.

Medication, can, however, act as an enabler, helping you or your child slow down, and be receptive to and able to adopt a structure that improves organization.

1. Medication Does Not Make the Individual Organized.

Organization is a skill that is taught, initiated, and repeated. While medication has benefits, the ADHD individual must learn and adopt lifelong habits to stay in touch with and to control his environment and belongings.

2. Medication Does Not Decrease Forgetfulness.

Since ADHD individuals are often forgetful, people assume they have bad memories. Memory actually does not appear to be a problem with most ADHD individuals. In fact, ADHD children seem to learn and recall information as well as their non-ADHD counterparts. However, since the ADHD individual is more distracted and impulsive, he may be less able to focus on the sequence of actions that must be completed. Medication will not help a child remember his homework, book bag, or glasses, but he may *seem* less forgetful, so people assume his memory has improved. Medication might slow down the flight of ideas, allowing him to learn organizational skills.

3. Medication Does Not Create or Teach the Routines
That Overcome Problems That Plague ADHD Sufferers.

It won't get your son up on time in the morning or teach your daughter how to organize her notebooks. One young man showed remarkable improvement on medication. He was much less distractible on Ritalin and able to record all of his homework assignments. He was able to bring home the correct books to complete those tasks most of the time. But Ritalin didn't teach him to put his homework in the correct folder or in his book bag, so he still had trouble finding the papers he had diligently completed the night before. And as hard as it is to believe, while he was an excellent musician, he is still the only kid we've met who was able to misplace his cello!

However, once his parents recognized that organizational difficulties still hampered Ben's success, most of the problems were overcome. Medication helped Ben be more receptive to help and more able to follow through on a task. Places at home were identified for his book bag, cello, and other items. New spiral notebooks with pockets where Ben could put each night's homework for each class were purchased. One by one, routines were created and introduced to overcome each problem.

Most ADHD adults recognize and crave the benefits organization will bring. Children are often too young or immature to recognize how much their own behavior contributes to their workload. Motivating the child to adopt routines often requires the use of outward incentives until the payoffs are felt.

WHAT ELSE YOU MUST DO

Most people who are organized have a system—or a number of systems—they employ to stay organized. To become organized you must recognize a need, adopt a place for the pieces, and break the tasks into a completable sequence.

Over the years we've noted recurring themes as we work with ADHD children and adults. A number of obvious problems might sound familiar to you:

- Getting up and getting dressed.
- Being punctual.
- Forgetting or losing things.
- Using time wisely to complete a task.
- Being overwhelmed by a task.

A number of these problems could be solved by adopting specific routines designed to alleviate each one. In the rest of this chapter we will present some solutions to common problems—solutions that many of the ADHD adults and children we've worked with created. In so doing, we're not putting ourselves at risk, because the most successful routines are ones designed by the people who will use them. That's one of the major reasons why the routines we'll present have worked!

With each of these individuals, we worked through a process to discover the right solution. As you or your child works to solve a problem and make a routine a positive habit, keep these suggestions in mind too.

IDENTIFY A PROBLEM

If it has happened three or more times, it's time to call it a problem. Stop!

By this point you're probably saying to yourself, "If getting myself (or my child) to follow a routine were easy, I would have done it years ago." We've put to use a little gimmick that has helped a number of ADHD children and adults adopt routines to overcome habitual problems. It's called *STOP*. It's an easy-to-learn, simple mnemonic to jog your memory to solve a recurring problem. You might prefer to call it an "Uh-oh" response. For us, STOP is a jump start for getting organized:

Stop
To
Organize the
Problem

DESIGN A ROUTINE TO OVERCOME THAT SPECIFIC PROBLEM

The routines we present are sample solutions. They may or may not match your individual needs or style. We've found that children are especially creative in solving a problem once the need is clearly identified. This is especially true if you "join the child" in problem solving. Saying, "You know, we have a problem. This week you did an excellent job on your homework, but it never got to your teacher. We need to find a way to get your homework to school every day," is much better than, "You left your homework at home every day this week. That's ridiculous." Couching the issue in terms of "*We* have a problem" prevents the feeling that it's you *against* the child or spouse. Instead, it is framed as being you *and* the individual against the problem.

Most people view getting organized as an overwhelming task, because we tend to think of "getting organized" as one HUGE undertaking. However, each day is composed of many routines. When you break them down, you usually end up with a series of activities that fall into some logical sequence. They may relate to the time of day or a sequence of tasks to complete a larger job. Tying a routine to a time or an event will make it easier to recall.

Looking at a day in the life of someone who is ADHD, it's easy to identify particularly troublesome routines.

A.M. Routines	*P.M. Routines*
Getting up	Doing Homework
Getting dressed	Getting Ready for Bed
Remembering materials for school/work	Packing the book bag/briefcase
	Winding down to fall asleep

SIMPLY SOLVE THE PROBLEM

Any routine that creates more problems than it solves is not worth the effort. On the other hand, a very creative solution—no matter how silly it may seem to you or to others—is good if it works.

> TIMOTHY *was eleven when he came up with a solution for one morning problem. He decided he needed three alarm clocks, one next to the bed, one across the room, and one by the door. He set the first alarm twenty minutes earlier than he needed to get up, knowing he could hit the snooze button one time. The second alarm went off ten minutes later. And the third alarm, set to go off five minutes after the others, bellowed, "Wake up, sleepyhead. Don't sleep your life away!" in an Arnold Schwarzenegger–type voice. Timothy's brother thought this whole rigmarole was ridiculous, but so what? It worked for Timothy and ended years of battles over getting up on time!*

MAKE SUCCESSFUL ROUTINES HABITS

To encourage this, base your routine on three *R*'s that prompt the behavior: **R**emember, **R**epeat, and **R**emind. For example, brushing teeth typically happens several times a day at a certain place. Time and place can be triggers that cause the action to be repeated. The routine of brushing teeth is *remembered* after eating. So eating becomes the prompt that jogs the memory. It is *repeated* at particular times: after breakfast each morning, before leaving for school, for example. The more times an action occurs under the same set of circumstances, the more likely it will become a habit.

It's unlikely that anything that happens once in a while will become habitual. A reminder is something you can add to your routine as a failsafe measure. If all else fails, a sign on the bathroom mirror or back door, or an index card with a list of daily things to do can act as a *reminder* to complete the action. Remember, Timothy included three clocks in his routine so he could not ignore the reminders to get up.

OFFER POSITIVE REINFORCEMENT FOR BUILDING A HABIT

Changing behavior is difficult, and new habits take time to build. Respect every bit of success.

Often people have an all-or-nothing attitude about new behavior. As long as you're doing it, everything is great. Forget once, however, and it's all over; there's no use in trying. That's not the way new behavior works. When a baby is learning to walk, he slips and falls hundreds of times before he becomes an accomplished walker. Everyone slips up once in a while when adopting a new behavior. Here are a few reinforcement tips to keep in mind as you or your child learns a new routine.

Start Small.
If your child is working on writing each homework task in an assignment book, first reinforce him for bringing the assignment to and from school. Next, praise and reward him for writing down the assignments. Or if you are working on keeping your desk neater, praise yourself for organizing one drawer at a time.

Keep a Record of the Number of Days in a Row the Routine Is Followed.
Keeping a concrete record of the accomplishment is very important. You can mark it on a calendar, or make a chart for your child to see the number of days she remembered to take her homework to school. It will make a difference.

When the day comes that she forgets her homework (and it will), don't consider it a failure. Simply announce your child's "world's record" up to that point: "Wow, you've remembered to take your homework to school eight days in a row. That's a new world's record. Today you forgot. Tomorrow starts a new opportunity to build a new world's record." You can also say the same types of things to yourself.

Praise and Reward Your Child and Yourself for Building a New Habit.
Encourage your child to recognize the change the new routine makes: "Remember all the times you forgot your homework? Aren't you proud of yourself for remembering to take it to school? And think of all the homework you did not have to redo!"

GET ROUTINELY READY

Just like anything worth learning, getting organized takes time and practice. This is only more true with skills that don't come naturally. However, here are some ways to ease the learning along.

Model It.

Being disorganized is definitely one trait you don't want to pass on. A good time to model good organization skills is at a weekly family meeting. Here you have the opportunity to talk about the important events of the coming week, goals, and how you plan to accomplish them.

Put It On the List.

We're big believers in lists. Let's face it: Even if you didn't keep lists when you were young, you are definitely going to need them when you get past forty! So why wait?

Use a calendar or daily planner, an assignment pad, an index card, or a self-sticking note pad. Have the materials available so that you get into the habit of making lists of what you need to do. That will automatically help your child break large tasks into smaller ones. In addition, if you or your child should become distracted, the list offers a means of getting back on track.

Make Sure You and Your Child Have a Daily Calendar or Assignment Pad Where Personal Plans, Homework Assignments, Tests, and Other Due Dates Can Be Recorded.

This is an important way to keep track of important dates, assignments, and other tasks.

Consider High-Tech Reminding Devices.

There are now many devices that will remind you of anything and everything you need to do. If you or your child is a computer fan, an electronic calendar or a calendar/organizer on your computer may be just the thing you are looking for. It's high-tech enough to be motivating, so you'll be more likely to record appointments and to write yourself reminders.

Identify Places for Things.

When everything has a place, everything is more likely to end up in its place. Identify and even label places for blocks, balls, art materials, and anything else. At home and the office, identify places for common working needs. A well-stocked desk is a necessity when you have tasks to complete. Label the spaces and *always* put each item in its designated location. A little obsessive-compulsiveness is okay at this time. Part of being organized is having what you need when you need it.

Establish a Special Place for Book Bags, Lunches, Keys, Etc.

This is so important we give it a section to itself. These items are common morning perils. Everyone gets tenser and later when someone must look for her keys, his book bag, or her purse, or must return to the house to get a lunch bag. Define a specific place for each one to sit day in and day out.

An ideal spot for the book bag is outside the bedroom door. Once the child correctly packs the bag with homework, books, etc., it is placed *outside* the bedroom door for you to check before you go to sleep. Use this idea or find another spot for your briefcase or other materials you need for work.

Create a File Drawer for Your Child's Schoolwork.

It may be in the desk or in a crate. Label the files with school subjects, extracurricular activities, and other favorite topics, such as video games, Magic Cards, or whatever your child is "into." This way he learns early on how and where to put important papers that relate to a topic. He can keep old tests, course materials, calendars, and other helpful notices from becoming clutter.

Dump the Drawers.

Mess breeds more mess. Dump the contents of a drawer onto the floor and throw out everything that you don't need. Give each drawer a theme, from socks to sweaters, and staples to notebooks. Help your child begin with neat drawers. For things that don't fit in a dresser, be creative. Use hooks, hangers, and bins to unclutter the clutter.

Turnabout Is Fair Play.

As soon as children are old enough, it should be their turn to clean up their stuff. You helped identify the locations, but when it comes to spring cleaning, it will be more meaningful if they are in charge. You can assist, but that's all. Surprise spot checks should include rewards for increasing neatness.

Have a Weekend Box.

Should toys or clothes pile up, put them in the weekend box. Rather than having fun, the child must spend time on the weekend helping you do the laundry or putting away toys as the logical consequence of not remembering the routine.

Encourage Your Child to Have an Address and Telephone Book from an Early Age.

As children make a new friend or acquaintance, they can add the name. The entire family can also keep a family address book for overall organization for car pools, friends, teachers, etc.

Keep a Master Family Planner.

Everyone's big dates, special projects, and events should be listed. Attend without fail the first parent-teacher meeting of the year to learn the teacher's expectations and plans for the year. Many teachers designate, for example, Friday as spelling test day. Knowing what to expect and placing predictable events on the calendar is very helpful.

Limit the Things on a Desk.

Now that there's a place for everything, there's no need for clutter. Create a work environment that is comfortable, that doesn't have distractions, and that you feel matches your style.

ROUTINES THAT WORK AT HOME, SCHOOL, AND WORK

Routines are a key component and seem to help keep ADHD individuals on track. Remove the routine, add a new distraction or a new task, and ADHD children and adults have a difficult time adjusting. Here are some routines that have worked for the adults and children we work with.

Bedtime Routine

The evening hours are often very difficult for ADHD youth and adults. There's a lot to do before bedtime, and sometimes a winding-down period gets lost in the events. Building a bedtime routine into the flow of the evening will help you or your child get ready to fall asleep.

The first step is to set a designated bedtime. An obvious but overlooked key to knowing if the selected bedtime works is how you or your child feels and acts in the morning. Dragging out of bed and grumpiness can be indications of not enough sleep. Of course, some people are morning people and others are not. If you have difficulty knowing how many hours your child needs to sleep, or find yourself fighting other sleep problems, refer to our first book, *Good Behavior,* or other books in the Resources section for additional help.

For younger children it is helpful to have a visual model of the bedtime routine to control the flow of events. With a marker, divide a white paper plate into five wedges. Cut out a cardboard arrow and attach it to the center of the plate with a brad. Label each section with an appropriate bedtime routine activity such as bath time, story time, cuddle time, quiet talk, and bedtime. With this tool, you have a visual reminder that will help you work through the evening routine.

Adults rarely consider themselves as needing a bedtime routine. However, a winding-down period will help you also. Listening to music, reading, or doing the relaxation exercises suggested in Chapter 10 will help you clear your mind, relax your body, and get ready to sleep.

Getting Up and Dressed On Time
The important elements of an effective morning routine include:

- Gathering clothes and materials for school or office.
- Determining a schedule for wake-up, breakfast, and departure.
- Identifying consequences for not meeting the schedule.

Peter blew up about once or twice a week when his mother asked him to change clothes because he was dressed inappropriately for school. The mornings were unpleasant because Peter grumped when his parents repeatedly prompted him to hurry, get dressed, and get downstairs. Even when Peter arrived downstairs in time to grab something to eat, he usually got angry when his sister reminded him that they needed to leave by 7:15 to get to school on time. As a result, Peter usually yelled, "I don't have time to eat," and left without eating, which added to his grumpiness. That also left his mother feeling guilty about sending him to school hungry.

In a session with the entire family, Peter accepted responsibility for his morning routine. It was agreed that he would lay out his school clothes the night before. Getting ready for bed would serve as the memory jogger to prompt him to lay out his clothes and put his book bag by the bedroom door. Mom had to okay the clothes the night before or accept the choice the next morning.

To aid the morning routine, Peter identified a wake-up schedule that worked for him. Ironically, it was suggested that he might be getting up too early in the mornings, and then dawdling away the excess time to such a degree that he was perpetually late. Instead, Peter decided to set a later wake-up time so he could sleep a little later. He identified the latest time he could arrive in the kitchen for breakfast, understanding that if he missed that time, breakfast would be placed in a brown bag to be eaten in the car.

Departure time remained 7:15 A.M., and Peter's sister agreed not to announce a countdown of the remaining minutes. In return, Peter understood that the car pool would pull out at 7:15 on the dot. If he missed the departure time, he would be unable to go to school that day and would remain in his room to write letters to each of his teachers explaining his absence.

This routine worked for Peter. His parents held their breath a number of mornings, agonizing about the possibility that he might miss the departure, but he never has.

Getting Out and About Without Leaving Anything

You've designated a place for everything, so how come you still get to the car without your keys, glasses, or notebook? Both children and adults can benefit from a little preventive medicine.

Before leaving home, work, the classroom, office, etc., do the *hesitation response*. Take a moment to make sure you have everything you need. First do a *body scan,* mentally covering your body from head to toe, making sure you have your hat, glasses, retainer, wallet, sweater—anything that relates to your personal needs.

Next, take a moment for a *mental scan* to review the day's schedule. Where are you going? What will you need? Do you have everything necessary for the day? If you can't trust your memory, review the day's events on your calendar, your daily planner, or an index card where you list them.

Finally, *scan the environment* to make sure you have taken your book bag, lunch, keys, purse, and anything else you have forgotten. Always ask yourself the key question before leaving a location: *"What have I forgotten?"*

A simple reminder is in order here. The hesitation response works best when you assign specific "homes" to objects you need every day.

After all, it does no good to scan the environment to jog your memory to take the keys, if the keys are not on the hook where they are supposed to be. The first routine should be practicing placing the items that are often forgotten, lost, or misplaced in the designated spots.

Getting Home with Everything You Need

The hesitation response is just as important when you leave a location. It's the last thing your child should do before leaving school each day. First he should scan his body for his hat, gloves, glasses, and jacket. Next he should look at his assignment book and make sure he has all the materials and books needed to complete his homework. Third, he should do a double check by scanning the environment to make sure he has taken all his belongings and has everything he needs for the night's tasks.

Keeping Tasks from Becoming Overwhelming

Many afternoons ten-year-old Janice would become overwhelmed by the homework that awaited her. When she got into the habit of *breaking the task into manageable pieces,* she felt less overwhelmed. With her parents' help, they defined a homework time. Janice wanted a break after school, so they decided she would play or watch television and begin homework at 4:30 P.M.

Helping Janice learn how to break her assignments into manageable pieces took more time and supervision. First, she decided to list each task on an index card. With her mother's help, she placed a line between items she felt she could do in one sitting. She also decided it would be a good idea to check off each task as it was completed. Between tasks, Janice set a five-minute timer so she could take a break. When the buzzer went off she returned to work.

Janice learned to use the same routine for any task that felt overwhelming. She listed each of the jobs involved, drew lines to identify activities she would do at one time, and rewarded herself with a break between them. She included checks on her own behavior by using a timer and checking off each completed task.

Learning to Be Punctual

One family we worked with struggled to be on time. The parents solved the problem by routinely setting ahead all the clocks in the house so as not to be late for anything. They also made it a habit to orally identify the times they had to be somewhere, the designated departure time, and the time to begin getting ready. The routine of always working backwards to identify a schedule for getting ready became a key element in the family's eventual punctuality.

An innovative adult creatively used his answering machine to keep himself on time. Interspersed amidst the voice mail from others, he left his own voice messages of things he needed to remember and places he needed to be. When he called in for his messages, the reminders prompted his behavior.

PUTTING ROUTINES TO WORK FOR YOU

It's your turn now. We've given you a method and suggested a number of routines that work for others. Try this assignment to identify a common organization problem and adopt a solution to correct it. At the end of the section you will find a work sheet you can use to create and track your own routines.

STOP.

Name one organizational problem that you or your child repeatedly has. **S**top **T**o **O**rganize the **P**roblem.

Identify the Time, Materials, or Event Involved in the Problem.

Does it occur at a particular time of day or in conjunction with an event? Are there particular materials involved? For example, eleven-year-old Sarah couldn't seem to remember to take her Ritalin. Her mother reminded her, but several mornings her Mom had to chase the car pool or take the medication to school. After that occurred several times, it was time to STOP.

We talked with the family about the problem. Sarah recognized the importance of taking her medication each morning. The behavior was tied to the household's morning hustle and bustle.

Create a Logical Sequence of Actions That Jog the Memory and Cause the Action to Occur.

For some children, breakfast is a natural memory jogger, but that hadn't worked for Sarah. Sarah decided to put the pills next to her toothbrush, because she did brush her teeth after breakfast. (She had braces and couldn't stand anything stuck in her teeth, so toothbrushing was one habit that caused no problems.) She wrote a rule for the routine: *Always take my pill before brushing my teeth,* and posted it on the mirror in the bathroom. She also put a sign on the inside of the front door, DID YOU TAKE YOUR MEDICINE? to remind her in case she had forgotten to take her medication.

Build the Habit.

It's hard work to build a new habit, so we gave Sarah a small calendar on which she could place an *X* each day she remembered to take her pill. The number of days in a row that she remembered became her "record to beat." Her parents then rewarded her each time she established a "new world's record" for the number of days in a row she remembered to take her medicine.

Stop

Name the needed routine:

_____

What materials are involved?

_____

Can you tie it to a time of day or an event?

_____

What event can you use to jog the memory to start the routine?

_____

What are the steps in the routine that will be repeated?

1. _____

2. _____

3. _____

What fail-safe measure can you implement to remind yourself?

_____

How will you keep track of the number of times you or your child follows the routine?

_____

How will you or your child be rewarded for solving this problem?

_____

A FINAL WORD

Most people find getting organized difficult. The difference is that whereas most people can get away with being disorganized, those with ADHD cannot. Since ADHD people are easily distracted, disorganization can "do them in." Being organized is a key to remaining in control and on-task. Medication cannot teach an ADHD child or adult how to be or stay organized. He or she must make this a long-term goal.

10

TAMING THE TIGER WITHIN

Cultivating Inner Calmness

BRIAN's parents chose not to put him on medication when they learned he was ADHD. He was not hyperactive and had never been accused of being a behavior problem in school. The family worked hard to help Brian keep up with his schoolwork and stay on top of things. He was in a structured school that was willing to make accommodations in the curriculum.

When Brian was in eighth grade, his parents noticed that he had begun biting his nails, and—as is typical of many adolescents—his mood fluctuated like the stock market. The family decided it was time to return to the clinic for additional help.

During therapy sessions, Brian was taught deep-muscle relaxation techniques and was encouraged to practice them diligently. To support the effort, we made a tape of the relaxation exercises, and Brian and his dad practiced them every evening. Both father and son became devoted advocates of the techniques. Brian reported that he could use the mini-relaxation exercises he learned to calm himself when he began to feel angry or anxious and before tests. His father used the relaxation techniques to fall asleep at night and to unwind after a stressful day at work.

Whether you are ADHD or not, learning techniques to calm yourself will help you manage the difficult times of the day and be the kind of person you want to be more often. Learning how to relax may be the greatest gift you ever give yourself or your loved ones if you are ADHD, or your child if she is ADHD.

Many different adjectives have been associated with ADHD, but *calm* is certainly not among them. Younger children who are hyperactive are described as "perpetual motion machines," or are accused of having "ants in their pants." For them, trying to sit calmly for any length of time is a real strain.

Adults frequently tell ADHD youngsters to "calm down." Unfortunately, this is something that they don't know how to do. Although a hyperactive child might be able to inhibit movement for a little while, the inner feelings of restlessness persist. Even during sleep their activity doesn't subside. The ADHD child's bed is often a knotted disarray of twisted sheets. Awake, many of these youngsters are easily excited by events around them. They have trouble suppressing reactions to others or avoiding being riled by changes in routines or unexpected events.

While many teenagers and adults with ADHD outgrow some of their outward hyperactivity, most continue to describe feeling squirmy, restless, and uneasy, so that experiencing calm would be a strange encounter indeed. Contending with the many problems related to ADHD often leaves them feeling anxious and agitated.

At its heart, ADHD is a problem of controlling physiological arousal. In fact, if you have ADHD, then it's quite likely the thought of relaxing and doing nothing drives you up the wall. For the ADHD child, the notion may be even more peculiar. However, to successfully manage the disorder, you or your child must find a means to calm the "tiger within."

WHAT MEDICATION CAN DO

When children, adolescents, or adults with ADHD have a very positive response to medication, their outward behavior often dramatically changes. Especially children, but older "good responders" too, become less fidgety and are able to sit still longer. The medication can lead to less impulsiveness, so they are less likely to blurt out thoughts and interrupt others. Their performance on objective computer tests such as the Gordon Diagnostic System, Test of Variable Attention (TOVA), and Conners Continuous Performance Test (CPT) also shows fewer impulsive errors. When the medication is "working," they seem more reflective and less quick to react to negative encounters or unanticipated occurrences. All of these changes in overt behavior make a good responder appear more calm. In short, medication can:

- Decrease overall activity level.
- Increase ability to sit still longer.
- Decrease impulsivity.
- Decrease reactivity.

WHAT MEDICATION CANNOT DO

Most people assume that if medication makes people look calmer, they must also feel calmer. Ironically, many children and teenagers who appear to respond well to medication report little change in how they actually feel. Instead, when asked about their responses to medication, they describe the transformation in terms of what they are able to accomplish or do better. After starting Ritalin, Matt said, "I know it's working because I can take the best notes I've ever taken. I can listen better." Carlene, a second-grader, proudly displayed her morning work to us and said, "I finished my work for the first time this year!" Even though their parents and teachers rated each of these children as being less fidgety, neither said he or she felt different.

These responses aren't unusual. Even those youngsters whom we recognize as being overmedicated and acting "zombielike" note little difference, offering only that they feel "weird." A child or adolescent may say he is tired or doesn't feel like talking to friends, but we can't recall a child describing himself as "calmer" or "more relaxed."

Adults too avoid labels like "calmer." They suggest they are in more control—at least for parts of the day. It is as though *calm* is not a word in their vocabularies.

Those individuals with less dramatic responses to medication frequently show little or no reduction in overt fidgetiness. Others exhibit some improvement in attention but very little decrease in activity level or impulsivity. On medication, these individuals neither appear nor report feeling "calmer."

It is fairly obvious, then, that the individual with ADHD does not feel calm. Moreover, regardless of what type of responder you or your child is, there are important things about being relaxed that medication does not teach. In short, medication does not:

- Teach the ADHD individual how to counter the stresses caused by ADHD.
- Teach the ADHD individual how to deal with anxiety.

- Teach the ADHD youth or adult how to counter anger.
- Teach the ADHD individual how to relax enough to enjoy quiet times.
- Teach the ADHD individual how to relax the body and mind enough to get to sleep more easily.
- Teach the ADHD individual how to deal with transition periods or rebound effects.

WHAT ELSE YOU CAN DO

If medication is not the answer to feeling relaxed, then whether or not you or your child takes medication, there are techniques to learn that promote calmness. In Chapter 11, "Alternative Treatments," we discuss the positive effects of biofeedback to calm the body. Even without biofeedback you can learn relaxation exercises to teach to your child or to calm yourself.

There is growing evidence that many ADHD youngsters differ from their regular classmates on a number of measures of tension and physiological arousal. Studies have shown that progressive relaxation training can lead to a decrease in tension and in some of the primary symptoms associated with ADHD. However, relaxation training may be even more impressive in helping to regulate what Drs. Keith Conners and Karen Wells, in their book *Hyperkinetic Children,* call the secondary symptoms of ADHD. These include explosive behavior, aggression, emotional ups and downs, and the feelings of lowered self-worth that often follow these reactions.

A child or adult who struggles with ADHD needs whatever help is available to counter the stress, anxiety, and frustrations she experiences. In addition, as a parent, partner, or friend of someone with ADHD, you have just as much need to remain calm—maybe more. Reacting to the crises that often accompany ADHD only escalates most situations. Mastering relaxation techniques provides you with the opportunity to remain calm amid turmoil as you model these skills for your child or spouse.

We feel so strongly about the benefits of relaxation skills that we have included chapters teaching relaxation exercises in each of our parenting books and in those devoted to ADHD. To develop your relaxation response and find more inner calm, practice the following steps.

STEP 1. LEARN DIAPHRAGMATIC BREATHING.

Research has shown that *how* you breathe affects not only your body but also your state of consciousness. When we are tense or upset, we tend to breathe in short, shallow "chest breaths." How do you breathe? Take a moment to place one hand on your chest and the other on your belly button. Breathe normally. Which hand rises more? If you are taking chest breaths, then your top hand is the one that is moving more. However, if you breathe through your diaphragm, the hand on your belly button is rising. Now place your hands around your waist. If you are taking full diaphragmatic breaths you should feel the sides at your waist also expand. Interesting, isn't it? Watch your child or spouse: How does he or she breathe?

Chest breathing raises the oxygen level and alkalinity of the blood to prepare us for what is referred to as the "fight or flight" response. An important part of our survival heritage, such breathing strategies ready the body to fight or flee an immediate danger. Like our cave-dwelling ancestors, we undergo profound physiological changes that protect us.

When an individual continues breathing in brief, shallow breaths for more than a few minutes, he is likely to experience a number of symptoms that interfere with concentration and that prompt stronger emotional reactions. Typically labeled as hyperventilation, rapid chest breathing leaves the individual feeling light-headed, as the oxygen levels in the brain increase. You may become aware of a tightening in the chest, or experience a tingling in the hands and legs. Commonly associated with panic or anxiety attacks, these symptoms are part of the activation of the sympathetic nervous system. Over time they lead to fatigue and more irritability.

Diaphragmatic breathing is calming. Babies do it naturally; opera singers do it on purpose. When you breathe through the diaphragm, you slow the body's physiological responses to stress.

To learn how to breathe through the diaphragm, get into a comfortable position. You may choose to recline in a comfortable chair or lie on the bed or floor. Rest your arms lightly by your sides. As you did when you were assessing how you normally breathe, place one hand on your chest and the other on your belly button. Take slow, easy breaths so the abdomen rises slowly. As you slowly inhale, count to five. The abdomen should rise as it inflates. If you or your child has difficulty sitting and doing this, try lying on the bed or on the floor. You may also place a book on the stomach area to encourage belly breaths.

As you exhale, slowly count to five and repeat to yourself the word *relax*. Pairing the word with exhaling will help the word become a future prompt for the relaxation response. Gradually increase the count as you exhale so that exhaling lasts longer than inhaling.

STEP 2. LEARN PROGRESSIVE-MUSCLE RELAXATION

Deep-muscle, or progressive-muscle, relaxation exercises offer some help in reducing the tenseness that individuals of all ages with ADHD experience. Progressive-relaxation training was first developed by Dr. Edmund Jacobson in the 1930s. It involves a series of sequential exercises in which various muscles of the body are systematically tensed and relaxed. Each muscle group in turn is relaxed until the entire body is in a state of equilibrium.

The advantages of deep-muscle relaxation exercises are likely to be obvious to you, but to your child they are not. As with most things that are good for you, your child is less likely to recognize the benefits of practicing these exercises. You will certainly want to practice them with your child, and perhaps increase the likelihood of your child's cooperation with a little reinforcement.

A brief description of deep-muscle relaxation exercise follows. The instructions can be easily modified to appeal to the younger child. Practice the techniques alone and then with your child so she can follow your model.

When doing the relaxation exercise with youngsters, you may describe tightening the limbs as making "arms of steel" or letting go as making "spaghetti arms" to illustrate tension versus limpness.

1. Get comfortable.
Have your child sit in a comfortable chair or recline.

2. Encourage the mood by faking a yawn.
First, pretend to yawn, opening your mouth wide and wrinkling your eyes. Inhale deeply through your mouth; then suddenly exhale, letting your face relax and your mouth close partially. Tell your child to open her mouth wide, breathe in a deep breath, and exhale, just as though she were yawning. Repeat the yawning routine several times, praising the performance. This isn't just being silly. Notice how faked yawns are followed by a few real ones.

3. Practice diaphragm breathing for a few minutes.

Repeat the exercises you learned previously. Make sure your child is comfortable doing "belly breathing" before beginning instruction in deep-muscle exercises.

4. Shrug the shoulders.

Instruct your child to lift her shoulders to her ears and hold them there as she inhales and counts to five. (Be sure she does not lift the shoulders too far or strain any muscles.) Have her exhale and say the word *relax* slowly to herself as she allows her shoulders to fall back into place. Repeat this exercise three times.

5. Relax the arms.

Have your child make a fist with one hand and slowly raise and extend the arm with closed palm down. Hold the position. Instruct her to take a deep breath and slowly count to five. At five, she opens the hand and drops the arm by her side as she whispers to herself the word *relax*. Repeat the exercise three times, alternating arms. When they are doing the exercises correctly, some people experience warm, tingly sensations and feelings of heaviness in the arms.

6. Loosen the legs.

(If you have back problems or if these exercises cause discomfort, stop and talk with your physician before practicing them.) Instruct your child to tighten the muscles in her left leg, making it stiff, and then lift it off the floor. Have her hold the position as she inhales and counts to five. At the count of five, instruct her to exhale and drop the leg to the floor as she whispers the word *relax*. Repeat the exercise three times on each side, alternating legs.

7. Flex the feet.

Have your child flex her feet, so that her toes point toward her head. Direct her to maintain the flex as she inhales and counts one, two, three, four, five. At five, have her release her feet and exhale, saying the word *relax* to herself. Repeat three times.

STEP 3. LEARN HOW TO MEDITATE.

Meditation is more than a fad. The positive effects of meditation are known by millions of people and have been practiced for centuries. However, you don't have to go to India, memorize a mantra, or wangle an introduction to the newest guru to learn this valuable technique. Dr. Herbert Benson of Harvard University introduced the *relaxation response* in his book of the same name in 1975. Dr. Benson's book recently has been republished, and you may find the techniques quite valuable.

The technique introduced by Dr. Benson has been shown to lower blood pressure and alter physiological measures that can have significant effects on health. While it may be harder for a person with ADHD to concentrate on these techniques, we have known many who benefited from practicing them.

STEP 4. ADD IMAGERY TO THE ROUTINE.

It might seem strange that people have to learn how to relax. But, like anything else worth doing, relaxation skills take time and practice to learn. You will find that over time, your mind will help ready your body to relax. You may enhance the effect by using visual imagery. After practicing belly breathing, and still lying in a comfortable position, imagine a favorite scene such as lying on warm sand at the beach as the waves lap the shore. Lie there basking in the image before continuing. You may want to use environmental audiotapes to aid your imagination.

Children can also use visual imagery to enhance the effects of deep-muscle relaxation. At the beginning of the exercises, after belly breathing, or at the end, describe in soft melodic tones the following images or others that you create of places the family has visited. Record them on an audiotape for your child to use when you are not available:

Imagine you are lying on the beach at _____ where we went _____ . It's a quiet afternoon after an active morning at the beach and your body is ready to relax. You're lying on the warm sand, and the hot sun is beating down on you. You feel its warmth and you hear the sounds of the ocean lapping the shore as the waves come in and out, in and out. You hear the sound of the gulls flying overhead and the waves continue to go in and out, as they make their path along the shore. . . .

You can also use positive imagery to help your child feel more confident in stressful situations. Once your child has mastered the relaxation techniques, create scenes for visual imagery in which your child sees himself performing well in a particular situation. For example, Caroline became very anxious about tests. She studied hard and worked to develop a variety of techniques to keep herself on track during tests. However, she worried so much about becoming distracted that she developed test anxiety and panicked on several quizzes. To counteract her fears, her parents helped her practice the relaxation exercises. Once she was able to relax herself, they taught her to visualize herself remaining calm and completing a test. After Caroline practiced her deep-muscle relaxation skills, her mother led her through an imaginary scene in which Caroline felt herself tense during a test, practiced belly breathing, and was able to calm herself. After a number of such sessions, Caroline reported that she did not panic on her history quiz and was able to complete all of the questions.

STEP 5. PRACTICE RELAXATION REGULARLY.

Not only must you and your child both practice the relaxation techniques, you also need to use them. At first, practice once a day; then move to several times a week. It's easy to incorporate the exercises into a nighttime routine, but you'll find them very helpful after school or work for winding down after a stressful day.

Prompt yourself and your youngster to practice relaxation skills with a simple chart. Often the simple act of keeping a public record of how many times each of you practices will keep the routine alive. Copy the chart in Figure 10.1 to keep track of the number of times family members practice relaxation skills. You may use the chart like a bar graph to keep a record of the number of times each week you or your child practices the relaxation exercises.

STEP 6. PRACTICE MINIRELAXATION EXERCISES
IN EVERYDAY SITUATIONS.

Many youngsters resist using relaxations skills, especially in public, for fear of looking silly. You may be able to overcome such reluctance by demonstrating ways to make it less noticeable. While sitting in the car or at a restaurant, instruct the youngster to simply tighten his grip on the arms of his chair and then relax, or to push his legs against the floor and then relax. Yawning and deep breathing can also be done quite inconspicuously.

Dr. Charles Stroebel invented a six-second relaxation technique that is quite effective. Copy the instructions shown below on a three-by-five card or your business card and keep them in your wallet. Use the technique frequently, especially when you are feeling tense or anxious.

1. Smile to yourself.
2. Clench your teeth slightly.
3. Inhale as you count to five.
4. Exhale and drop your mouth open slightly.
5. Feel the tension drain all the way to your toes.
6. Think to yourself, "Leave my body out of this."

Encourage your child to practice minirelaxation techniques when he finds himself in a stressful situation, such as before exams, during disagreements, or when he's bored. They are also helpful during the periods when medication is wearing off.

STEP 7. CREATE A MENU OF RELAXING ACTIVITIES.

Make a list of some of your favorite relaxing activities. These are likely to be enjoyable to anyone, but perhaps particularly important to ADHD individuals who cannot unwind in other ways. Add your favorites to the menu below.

■ Menu of Relaxing Activities

1. Soaking in a warm bath.
2. Listening to soft, melodic, music.
3. Stroking a pet.
4. _____
5. _____
6. _____

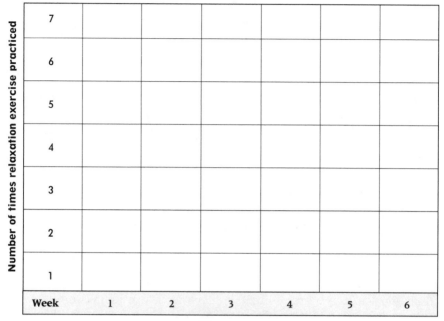

Figure 10.1
Relaxation Chart

A FINAL NOTE ON RELAXATION

By adding to your youngster's or your own repertoire of calming techniques, you gain a sense of control over your body and mind so that you feel you can manage your ADHD. It is not an illusion. The research increasingly indicates that the mind-body connection is much stronger than most of us realize. Relaxation exercises remain one of the best ways to manage the symptoms of ADHD and to permit the individual to acquire feelings of control.

11

ALTERNATIVE TREATMENTS

Fads, Fallacies, and Facts

Y ou've probably heard about the Feingold diet, and you're probably
quick to read any article that touts a remedy for ADHD. Perhaps a
friend tried amino acid therapy, another took her child off all sugars, and
your mother-in-law heard about biofeedback. You read about inner-ear
therapy for ADHD in a recent best-selling novel and wonder whether the
protagonist was right to extol the merits of this treatment. Should you
rush to try any one of these techniques?

Once you begin your search, you may be surprised to discover a
wide range of solutions offered by everyone from well-meaning friends
to unfamiliar proponents of the newest "off the beaten track" therapy.
However, there are no quick fixes for ADHD, and almost all of the remedies you hear about require time, effort, and, most often, money. Which
alternative treatments hold promise? Which ones should you try? Are
there any that are a waste of time? This chapter will help you make these
decisions.

JUDGING A NEW TREATMENT FOR ADHD

What criteria should you use to evaluate a treatment? Because it works
for Sam Jones or his son Alvin, will it work for you or your child? Even
effective treatments for ADHD are not equally beneficial for all children,
adolescents, and adults. Some treatments have been arduously tested by
well-designed and well-executed research; others may be instituted
without proof or strong support for the technique. Your guard should be

up for any treatment that seems to promise too much too soon. As you well know, ADHD is not a problem that can be solved quickly.

Here we will present some of the best-known alternative treatments for ADHD. Some, like the Feingold diet, have been used for years; others have a more recent origin. Some have proven merit, others hold promise, and still others may not be worth your time.

THE FEINGOLD DIET

In 1975 Dr. Benjamin Feingold suggested that children's behavior was influenced by the additives in food. In particular, he hypothesized that more than half of ADHD children display hyperactivity, inattentiveness, and other characteristics of the disorder because of the additives in the food they eat. Over time, Dr. Feingold and others refined the diet to exclude not only all additives but also artificial flavorings, food colorings, and preservatives.

People who believe in the Feingold treatment for ADHD are enthusiastic about its merits. Unfortunately, there is very little research evidence to support Feingold's initial claims. At best, a very small number of ADHD children may experience relief from such a healthy but strenuous diet.

Dr. Keith Conners, a well-respected researcher of ADHD, originator of the Conners Ratings Scales and author of *Feeding the Brain: How Foods Affect Children*, relates a very interesting experience that occurred when he and his colleagues tried to test the Feingold diet. For their test, they divided a group of children whose behavior dramatically improved when they were on the Feingold diet into two groups. One group received chocolate cookies that were made with artificial color; the second group received a placebo cookie, identical to the first except that it contained no artificial colors. In addition, neither the researchers nor the parents knew which group got which cookie. It was impossible for the children to tell the difference between the cookies, since they tasted the same.

A very hyperactive seven-year-old child in the test improved dramatically on the Feingold diet. However, after this boy ate one cookie, his mother frantically called Dr. Conners with the news that the child had "gone wild," wielding a knife and wreaking havoc! Since it was a double-blind study, no one knew which cookie the child received until the envelope containing that information was opened. The fact was, this child had received a placebo cookie. His abrupt behavior change was not caused by additives at all! Further, when the study was concluded, the overall effects did not indicate that additives significantly affected the children's behavior.

Keeping a child on the Feingold diet is a remarkable challenge. Those parents and children who succeed have certainly learned how to manage some aspects of their behavior. However, the changes in behavior that result are not likely to be caused by the lack of particular substances in the child's diet.

SUGAR INTAKE AND HYPERACTIVITY

Many parents report a direct correlation between hyperactivity and their children's consumption of sugar. When their child eats some candy, he is wild; no sugar, and all is better. In those households, Halloween is the most reviled holiday.

The sugar-ADHD connection has some plausibility. One of the strongest explanations for ADHD rests on the assumption that certain neurotransmitters in the brain control alertness, activity, and arousal. Two transmitters in particular are considered to play a role in ADHD: dopamine and norepinephrine. Usually their coordination is sympathetic, but in ADHD it is not. It is thought that one reason medications affect ADHD behavior is that stimulants, for example, help to resynchronize the action of the neurotransmitters.

Food sources undoubtedly play a role in the production of certain neurotransmitters. Certain proteins found in food contribute to this development. Sugar may sometimes help certain proteins get to the brain, while on other occasions sugar is thought to prevent that link.

Dr. Ronald Prinz of the University of Florida undertook a study of children's reaction to sugar in 1980. Ninety-one four- and five-year-olds, some of whom had daily diets containing more than twice the adult consumption of sugar, were included in the study. Dr. Prinz found that children with a high intake of sugar had lower attention spans. Other studies have found a high correlation between aggressive behavior and sugar intake.

Dr. Jane Goldman at the University of Connecticut has also studied preschoolers' reaction to sugar. Using a continuous-performance task of the type often used with ADHD youngsters, she compared the children's performance after drinking a sugar drink or a placebo without any sugar. After one hour, Dr. Goldman found a definite decline in the performance of the children who drank the sugar drink. The children made almost twice as many errors after they drank the sugar drink as when they drank the placebo. They also engaged in more hyperactive behavior and less on-task behavior during a period of one hour to one and a half hours after drinking the sugar drink. Before or after this time period, few differences in behavior were noted.

Still, the evidence about children's response to sugar remains far from clear. Other studies have come to different conclusions. One study conducted by Keith Conners documented children's intake twenty-four hours a day for six months. Part of the time, one group received additional sugars. The researchers were able to keep an exact record of what each child ate because the children were all patients in a psychiatric ward—which certainly adds another kind of "food for thought" to this study. The results of this study showed that, on the average, children were slightly less active on sugar days than on placebo days! However, these days also coincided with occasions when the children's breakfast included higher protein levels. If the children ate eggs, meat, fish, or cheese, the additional sugar was beneficial. When their breakfast had a higher sugar level compared with the level of protein, the additional sugar coincided with greater activity.

Additional research supplies more information. Following a trail to determine why children react differently to sugar in their diet, some research appears to indicate that hyperactive children produce more of the hormone cortisol after eating sugar. This is contrary to what occurs in normal children. Since cortisol is the hormone produced by the body during a stressful event, it may in fact play a role in the children's behavior.

Obviously, the research is not conclusive about the effect of sugar in the diet. It is quite likely there is not a singular effect, in any case. The rest of the child's diet, the age of the child, what he eats for breakfast, and individual characteristics are likely to affect the outcome. However, at the present time there is no justification for removing sugar from a child's diet. A well-balanced diet is probably still the best approach to avoiding any extreme influences related to food.

AMINO ACID THERAPY

The brain and body need particular nutrients to function. These most often are chemicals that the body does not produce itself. For example, the brain has neurotransmitters that act as chemical communicators in the brain. Amino acids play an important role in the production of certain neurotransmitters, including those that have a role to play in ADHD.

The theory that a lack of certain amino acids may affect the production of certain neurotransmitters has substance. Some amino acids cannot be produced by the body and so must be supplemented by diet. When the body cannot produce these amino acids, we know it creates problems for the individual. Therefore, it would seem plausible that ADHD is caused by the absence of certain amino acids. At least the theory looks pretty good on paper. However, studies have not upheld it. There is no evidence that amino acid treatment helps children with ADHD. Don't count on it to solve your child's problems.

MEGAVITAMINS AND MINERAL SUPPLEMENTS

Many people believe if a few vitamins are good for you, a lot of vitamins are great. We know that specific vitamin deficiencies can cause certain illnesses; an absence of vitamin D, for example, causes rickets. Given this bit of information, it is only a slight leap of logic to assume that large doses of vitamins and minerals might decrease hyperactivity and improve attention.

Although in the 1950s and 1960s vitamin therapy was used to treat some forms of mental illness, there is very little support for this approach for ADHD. Unfortunately, there is no evidence from well-designed studies that supports such a notion. In addition, overdoses of certain vitamins can be harmful.

ANTIMOTION MEDICATION

Many children who are diagnosed with ADHD have problems with gross motor skills and coordination, and are generally awkward and clumsy. Perhaps this is the basis of a recent theory that ADHD is caused by a problem in the inner ear. Dr. Harold Levinson, in his book *Total Concentration: How to Understand Attention Deficit Disorders, Maximize Your Mental*

Energy, and Reach Your Full Potential, puts forth the theory that the inner ear regulates balance, voluntary movement, and the body's energy levels. Dr. Levinson postulates that a disturbance in this system causes "sensory scrambling," which means the brain is unable to shut out distracting sensory input, causing ADHD, reading problems, and other difficulties.

Dr. Levinson, who claims to have evaluated more that twenty thousand people with ADHD and other learning disabilities, suggests that ADHD and dyslexia can be treated with antimotion pills in combination with a variety of other medications, including stimulants. In his book, he presents anecdotal support for his theories.

At present, though, no research substantiates any relationship between attentional processes and the vestibular system that controls motion and balance. Furthermore, there is no documented evidence from Dr. Levinson or others that antimotion pills improved ADHD or reading disabilities.

CANDIDA YEAST

Candida yeast lives in your body, your child's, ours, everyone's. That's normal. Sometimes when friendly bacteria are killed off by antibiotics, yeast can grow out of normal bounds. Women are familiar with this occurrence in the form of vaginal yeast infections. However, yeast infections also can occur on nails, on the skin, or in the mouth.

Dr. William Crook, author of *The Yeast Connection,* suggests that many, many problems—both mental and physical, and including ADHD—are caused by yeast. Dr. Crook does not explain how this occurs, but he does offer a treatment that includes a special diet, an allergy-free environment, medication for yeast, tutoring, positive discipline, and nutritional supplements of minerals and vitamins.

Although Dr. Crook reports the effects of his treatment on many youngsters, there is no research evidence to support his contentions about the yeast connection. There is no outside research evidence to support this theory and treatment approach.

CHIROPRACTIC

Neural organization technique is a chiropractic approach to the treatment of learning disabilities and ADHD. According to this theory, misalignment of certain portions of the skull and spine causes these problems. As the reasoning goes, spinal adjustments will correct the misalignment and cure the learning and attentional problems.

Chiropractic is a popular health-care option, but there is no research evidence in leading medical or psychological journals that chiropractic manipulations will cure learning disabilities or ADHD.

INTEGRATIVE SENSORY TRAINING

Dr. Jean Ayres, an occupational therapist, coined the term *sensory integration* to explain the brain's ability to organize stimuli and recognize information coming through all the senses. She suggests that many problems are caused by the brain's inability to integrate the myriad of information arriving through the senses. When this occurs, information is misinterpreted so that children may have problems with balance, motor planning, attention, and perception. As a result, individuals experience learning, attention, speech, coordination, behavioral, and social problems, and may be uncomfortable "in their own skins," very sensitive, or overwhelmed by stimuli.

Children with ADHD often have some of the problems Dr. Ayres discusses. They can be clumsy and become overwhelmed by stimuli. They also show characteristics of tactile defensiveness—finding clothes, socks, shoes, and other apparel unbearably uncomfortable. They may not like the feel of water on their faces or having their hair washed.

Dr. Ayres suggests sensory integration therapy to remedy these problems. One of the most commonly used exercises, "brushing," is designed to use the nerve-cell connections in the body to help the brain organize itself. With this technique, a very soft plastic-bristle brush is rubbed across the child's limbs and back, after which pressure is applied to the joints of the shoulder, knee, and hip.

Many children enjoy being brushed and participating in the other exercises designed for sensory integration. Whether these have a positive impact on ADHD is not shown, nor is it documented by well-controlled studies of ADHD youth.

BIOFEEDBACK/NEUROFEEDBACK

Proponents of EEG biofeedback claim that children who have attention deficit disorder are unable to concentrate because they have abnormal brain-wave patterns. Dr. Joel Lubar of the University of Tennessee is one of the best-known proponents of neurofeedback for ADHD. He believes that ADHD is a secondary symptom of an underlying neurological disorder. Specifically, individuals with ADHD have decreased arousal stemming from increased theta-wave activity in the frontal and central lobes of the brain. These slower theta waves are typically associated with daydreaming, in contrast to the faster beta waves usually associated with arousal and concentration.

Neurofeedback is a form of biofeedback, in which EEG biofeedback equipment is used to train individuals with these patterns to increase beta-wave production and inhibit theta-wave production to improve the youngster's or adult's ability to concentrate. Lubar has been working with neurofeedback for the treatment of ADHD for fifteen years. According to his research, many children treated with EEG biofeedback have been able to decrease their medication for hyperactivity by learning to control brain-wave activity.

A recent study on biofeedback holds promise. Published in 1995 in *Biofeedback and Self-Regulation,* the research study by Troy Janzen found that students ages eight to nineteen years old, after participating in a summer program of intensive neurofeedback training, were able to decrease theta-wave activity and show significant improvement in WISC-III scores following training. In addition, parent ratings improved following neurotraining.

However, not all the evidence is in on biofeedback training. It is an area of research that may hold valuable information. If you choose to proceed with this technique, use it in conjunction with a multimodal approach to treating ADHD, and work with a professional who is highly sophisticated in the use of neurofeedback to treat ADHD.

FINDING HELP

The grass always looks greener on the other side of the fence. Many out-of-the-mainstream therapies look promising, but few have stood up to well-controlled research.

The best-designed research indicates the best treatment for ADHD is a multimodal approach. This may at times include medication, classroom interventions, behavior modification, parent training, couples therapy, social-skills training, cognitive therapy, and family therapy. As you know, finding the right professional to orchestrate diagnosis and therapy is an important component of a successful outcome for you or your family.

As a parent or adult, you are ultimately responsible for the choice of therapies and for following through on whatever approaches you select. However, feeling comfortable with a therapist and the plan of action you have chosen is important.

FINDING A THERAPIST

Selecting a professional is often a frightening and bewildering experience. If you are a parent who has just been told your child may have such a problem, you'll be making difficult decisions about how to proceed and whom to trust.

Your goal should be to match your needs to the skills and expertise of the therapist. It's not always easy to make the match, but you increase your chances by doing your homework. The suggestions that follow are designed to help you find the person who can best provide you with the kind of help you need.

Get educated.

If this is the only book you've read on the subject, peruse others at your local bookstore or library. Attend a meeting of a support group for attention deficit disorder (see "Organizations and Support Groups That Can Help" in the Resources section).

Ask a doctor, friend, or school principal/counselor for suggestions.

Request from each the names of three candidates who fit your present needs and are known for their work with ADHD children or adults. Call your local chapter of the American Psychological Association, Learning Disabilities Association, or Children With Attention Deficit Disorder for professionals who specialize in ADHD in your area. Compare lists.

As you move through the process, collect the names of various people you hear about. You may work with one person for diagnosis and another for therapy. At different points in time, you may discover that you need to work with a different kind of specialist for a particular need. You may work with a psychologist for diagnosis and then interventions in the school. At a later date, your child might be ready for a social-skills class, so you would look for the appropriate course for that. If you elect to use medication, you must work with an M.D. who can prescribe medication. Depending on your situation, you may choose to work with a psychiatrist or continue to monitor the medication by combining the skills of your pediatrician or family physician and psychologist.

Decide on three to five professionals to interview, taking into consideration reputation, location, and area of expertise.

Some therapists will be glad to talk with you by phone; others will prefer you make an appointment, for which you will be expected to pay. In either case, feel free to discuss your concerns and ask your questions.

Ask a lot of questions.

Here are some suggestions:

1. How do you go about diagnosing ADHD?
2. How much experience and training do you have working with ADHD children (or adults)?
3. How do you usually work—with the child, with the family, in the school, etc.?
4. How do you feel about medication? How do you monitor medication? If the individual is not an M.D.: How will you work with a physician to prescribe medication?
5. What are the elements of treatment for ADHD?
6. What services do you offer in your office for ADHD youth, adults, families? For example, do you have a children's support group, social-skills training groups, specialized tutoring, etc.?
7. What is the cost per session for an individual, family, or group?

Once you have chosen someone to work with, continue to ask questions. When you have a diagnosis, ask for an explanation of particular characteristics. You will want to know if your child has additional learning problems. The psychologist who completes the psychoeducational evaluation should provide a written report that outlines test results, conclusions, and suggestions for treatment. Still, feel comfortable asking all the questions you need to understand how your child's or your own problems play out in daily life. In addition, make sure the components of the treatment plan are clearly presented.

Don't get overwhelmed.

There will be a lot of information to take in at once. Don't assume you or your child will be in constant treatment for life. There will be times when everything moves along smoothly, and you do not need ongoing therapy. At other times, there will be problems that require a more concerted effort and the support of a therapist. If you elect to use medication, drug therapy needs will change with growth and maturity. As you or your child learns the skills to compensate for various aspects of ADHD, you may also find that you need less or different kinds of help.

12

ADHD GROWN UP

From Disc Jockeys to Doctors

If you're a parent of an ADHD child, you probably worry a lot about how this disorder will affect your youngster when he grows up. Will he outgrow it? Will ADHD prevent her from succeeding in college and making her way in her chosen career? Might he experience more serious problems that have been associated in the press with this disorder?

If you're an adult diagnosed as ADHD, you want to know why you haven't outgrown this syndrome. You want to understand all of the ways ADHD is affecting you at work, at home, and in your interactions with others. Does it contribute to the feelings of depression you sometimes experience? Is it an explanation for your procrastination or frustration on the job? How does it influence your relationship with your spouse and children? Most important, you want to know what to do now to solve these problems.

We have heard hundreds of stories about what happens to ADHD children when they grow up and how adults with ADHD are managing. Some are genuine success stories; others are stories about struggling to avoid not-so-happy endings. Whether they become doctors or dropouts, write the great American novel or become the world's greatest salesperson, or are great parents or partners, what factors make the difference in the lives of ADHD adults? Why do some succeed and others struggle?

As research has verified that ADHD is not simply a childhood disorder, there has naturally been increasing interest in the effects of ADHD on adults. Adults who have long known that difficulties with attention, distractibility, and impulsivity persist past adolescence feel vindicated by the research: PET scans show differences in the brains of adults with and without the disorder. And as more and more adults are seeking and finding a diagnosis of ADHD for their troubling symptoms, support groups for adults with ADHD are springing up to console, inform, and support these individuals and their families.

As the facts emerge, adult interest in ADHD and the information we have about ADHD in adulthood converge in several important areas: Most people do not outgrow ADHD; medication is not a long-term cure for the disorder; and ADHD in adults is rarely an individual's only problem. However, the most important fact to know is that it is never too late to get help for ADHD.

YOU JUST DON'T OUTGROW ADHD

The conventional wisdom used to be that youngsters would outgrow ADHD after puberty. However, recent research has clearly established that for most people this is not the case. Although approximately half of the individuals correctly diagnosed with ADHD will experience significant decreases in hyperactivity, 20 to 65 percent of them will continue to have problems with impulsivity, distractibility, and inattention throughout their adult years.

Unfortunately, these persistent aspects of the disorder can cause the older teen and adult to have continuing difficulties in academics, as well as recurring social and behavior problems. Thus, while it has been suggested that 3 to 5 percent of all children, or one out of every twenty-five to thirty youths, have ADHD, it is estimated that approximately one out of every thirty-five adults still exhibits symptoms of the disorder in adulthood. These statistics translate into more than 2 million school-age children afflicted with ADHD and from 500,000 to 1 million adults whose daily lives are affected by the disorder.

As researchers and clinicians become aware of the great numbers of adults who were misdiagnosed or never diagnosed in childhood and adolescence, many are beginning to realize that our current estimates may be only guesses as to the actual number of children and adults with ADHD. In fact, there are those who think these numbers grossly underestimate the real dimensions of the problem.

Whatever the true incidence of ADHD in adulthood, the fact remains that for many people, ADHD is a lifelong condition that has a variety of faces, traits, and characteristics, most of which can adversely affect daily life. Most important, there are a number of points you must keep in mind as you help yourself, your child, or your spouse overcome the effects of this disorder.

MEDICATION TAKEN IN CHILDHOOD
DOES NOT HAVE A LASTING EFFECT

There have been a number of retrospective studies of the childhood of individuals diagnosed as ADHD as adults, as well as prospective studies that followed ADHD children as they grew into adulthood. In their book *Hyperactive Children Grown Up,* Drs. Weiss and Hechtman assimilate the findings of the longitudinal research on ADHD children grown up conducted between 1960 and into the 1980s at Montreal Children's Hospital and McGill University, as well as studies done elsewhere. Their conclusions indicate that even when children respond well to medication for a number of years, there is little detectable difference between those individuals and others who did not take medication. The key to positive outcomes among children treated for ADHD is not the adoption of drug therapy, but the inclusion of multimodal treatment, including educational interventions and counseling in a treatment effort lasting more than three years. Those individuals who received combined treatment were found to have fewer problems when they reached age nineteen and beyond than those young adults who did not. It is clear that although early diagnosis and intervention are important, treatment must be comprehensive and sustained to have a lasting effect.

MANY ADHD ADULTS HAVE A COMBINATION
OF PROBLEMS

By the time many people with ADHD reach adulthood, they have developed a number of other problems. This is especially true of those who have not had the benefit of treatment. Many have lowered self-esteem and a damaged self-concept. While most are gainfully employed, their job status is often inferior to that of their counterparts who do not have ADHD. In addition, adults with ADHD have a history of frequent job changes and do not reach their career goals as often. They also divorce more often and have more relationship problems.

Frequently, adults with ADHD experience other psychological problems as well. Often as a result of the struggles associated with ADHD, many of them suffer from anxiety and depression. They may have more basic anxiety disorders, mood disorders, and even thought problems that are not caused by ADHD. These coexisting, or so-called *comorbid*, conditions greatly complicate their lives.

Finally, there is evidence that, in contrast to their non-ADHD peers, adults with ADHD have a greater rate of alcohol and drug abuse as well as greater incidence of other addictions. Unfortunately, the problems with addiction may reflect the needs of untreated ADHD adults who are unknowingly attempting to self-medicate their ADHD symptoms. However, contrary to popular fear, there is no evidence these addictions are caused by taking stimulants or other medications as children. (See pages 17–18.)

While this may appear to be a depressing picture of ADHD outcomes, the current reality also points to an increasingly more positive future for those who are diagnosed with ADHD today. Information about ADHD has proliferated over the last twenty years. In the past, most children were not diagnosed with ADHD until they failed in school. One positive outcome of the increased press for ADHD has been earlier diagnosis, before children have failed in school or grappled and floundered so long with the disorder's negative characteristics that their skills suffer and their self-image is immeasurably tarnished. Furthermore, our increased understanding of the organic nature of the problem has had some positive results. It is now recognized as a disorder that threatens the positive future of individuals. The inclusion of ADHD in the Individuals with Disabilities Education Act (IDEA) means that the schools must provide appropriate education for children with this disorder, and that as a parent of an ADHD child, you have the right and obligation to be an advocate for your child. Furthermore, acceptance of ADHD as a disorder that threatens later success in adulthood hopefully mandates that money and efforts for research and treatment will be provided. Rather than children's being designated as dumb, having attitude problems, or being labeled inappropriately, it is recognized that ADHD children and adolescents have problems that require specific attention and treatment.

IT'S NEVER TOO LATE TO GET HELP

The adults we see who learn later in life that they are ADHD believe that years of problems and challenges could have been avoided or lessened if they had been properly diagnosed when they were children. However, it is never too late to get help. The following examples of two adults illustrate this point.

> Forty-year-old **SAM** was an ADHD adult diagnosed later in life. He was street smart and highly personable, but when he thought of his school years or his career, he clearly saw himself as a failure. Although good at sports, Sam never participated during high school or college because his low grades made him ineligible.
>
> "If I had only known as a kid what I know now, that I'm ADD, I might have been able to overcome some of my problems," Sam commented. "Everyone just said I didn't apply myself or use my potential, but no one ever said it wasn't my fault." Just knowing that he had a real, recognized condition relieved him of a great deal of guilt and pressure. Once Sam knew that he was ADHD, he was able to find appropriate professional help, including counseling, medication, and career consulting. Over a few years, Sam changed his career field into sports marketing, where his natural talents were appreciated and rewarded. In marketing and sales, his hyperactive nature was his greatest strength.

> In her early thirties, **MELISSA** was struggling to maintain a job and be a good wife and mother, but she felt herself slipping into a depression. She was irritable, always tired, and unable to participate in activities. As she described it to us, "I try to be everything for everyone, but I feel like the air is slowly leaking out of me." When she was diagnosed with ADHD, she was stunned. However, as she reminisced about her childhood and how distracted she was, everything seemed to come into focus.
>
> When Melissa first tried medication for ADHD, she felt like a new person, better able to deal with her sense of feeling overwhelmed all the time. However, medication was far from a cure-all. Knowing what was wrong helped Melissa to understand herself, but she still had to deal with years of low self-esteem and depression. Over time, with individual therapy and the help she found in a support group, Melissa became a much happier person.

There is much to learn from the experiences ADHD adults had growing up. Often they point out how a friend, a parent, a special teacher, or a therapist offered them support and understanding at key moments in their lives. The young adults we have worked with tell us how important it is for people to recognize that overcoming the effects of ADHD takes a variety of actions over the long haul.

Although many ADHD adults who were given medication as children express bitterness over their experiences, they also make it clear they did not understand why medication was prescribed. Often their reasons for disliking medication were totally unrelated to its effectiveness. Like the typical teenagers they were in many ways at the time, they were embarrassed by taking pills and hated feeling different. However, they remembered being told only that the pills would help them; they had little opportunity to understand the disorder, how it affected them, and why medication might help. In Chapter 5, we discuss how to present the idea of taking medication to your child so that future problems like these can be avoided.

Adults only recently diagnosed often tell us, "Just knowing I have ADHD finally gives a name to my problems other than laziness and stupidity." The diagnosis relieved guilt and provided a direction for their efforts.

Learning more about ADHD and what to do about each aspect of the disorder leads to finally being able to manage the troubling symptoms that have plagued progress. However, it is dangerous to assume that medication is the complete answer to ADHD. Understanding and treating each aspect of the disorder is as crucial for adults as it is for children.

WHAT MEDICATION CAN DO

If you took medication for ADHD as a child, you may have assumed that you had outgrown the medication along with the disorder. Neither may be true.

If you have been diagnosed as ADHD for the first time as an adult, you may assume that you are too old to take medication. That may not be true either.

A number of adults who responded to stimulant medication as children show similar responses when they take medication as adults. They may find they need larger dosages of medication to adjust for changes in weight, but many men and women are surprised to discover they respond well to smaller doses. Some individuals find that although they do not respond to stimulant medication, other types of medication such as antidepressants have a positive effect. Certain adults experience relief when they take a combination of medications.

Medication may improve many characteristics of ADHD. Understanding what medication can and cannot do for adult ADHD will give you a means to judge its effectiveness and determine what else you must do to cope with the effects of this disorder.

1. Medication Can Improve an Adult's Attention Span.

Many professionals have been pessimistic about the effects of medication on adults with ADHD and have resisted its use. However, studies of adults' response to stimulant medication report many adults treated with stimulants experience an increase in their ability to pay attention.

When an adult has a positive response to medication, it can increase his or her ability to concentrate longer and to complete tasks. Perhaps not surprisingly, the effect is similar to that seen in children. In a review of drug studies conducted with adults, Drs. Wender, Wood, and Reimherr found that 60 percent of adult patients diagnosed ADHD showed improvement with stimulant medication. While this is not as high a percentage of respondents as that seen with children, the positive effects are clearly strong and obvious.

Additional studies and a substantial number of clinicians report positive results with antidepressants and anticonvulsant medications such as clonidine. As with children, the responses to particular medications by adults seems to be very much an individual matter that requires monitoring by a skilled clinician. For more information about particular medications, refer to Chapter 5.

Over the past few years we have met a number of parents who, as they went through the evaluation process with their sons or daughters, began to see themselves in the diagnosis. For the first time they are able to put a name to the confusing collection of characteristics that has troubled them all their lives.

ALLEN *is a lawyer with a youngster whom we diagnosed with an attention deficit and who responded positively to stimulant medication. As Allen learned more about ADHD, he began to realize that he also had many of the characteristics of the disorder. Although he had trouble sustaining his attention long enough to read long passages, he had made it through college and law school by using friends' notes and working long hours with frequent breaks. Many an evening, the work that took others five or six hours required an overnight effort on his part. The same was true of his days as a lawyer. He found it difficult to sequence his work, especially in the afternoons. Finally, he asked to be tested for ADHD. With a confirmed diagnosis, his physician began him on a low dose of medication, 5 mg of Ritalin twice a day, assuming he would need to increase the medication to see an effect. Everyone was surprised by Allen's immediate response to medication. Suddenly, he was able to read entire contracts and organize his thoughts without getting distracted. He still had to be careful about when to schedule tasks that required the most concentration. However, medication made a major difference in his work effort.*

Forty-one-year-old FRANK *told his story at a support group meeting to illustrate the important role medication played in his life. ''As a child, I was a mess. No one knew what to do with me, and no one ever said it wasn't my fault. If I had only known what we know about ADHD today, I might have gotten the proper help. I still ultimately wish I didn't need medication,'' he commented. ''However, without it I couldn't write one page. I just can't seem to focus a complete thought without it, and Ritalin gives me the edge I need to accomplish this.''*

Frank was a struggling writer before medication. He was also an accomplished hair stylist. He chose the field of hair styling since it fit his personality and style completely. He didn't have to sit still, and with the quick turnover of clients, he felt repeated gratification and found success in his work. But his other dream of becoming a writer couldn't be accomplished without medication. It's a pleasure to report that Frank has had a number of articles published now in local and national magazines as he learns to ply his craft.

Both men's stories illustrate how, at least for these individuals, medication increased attention so that they could reach their career goals.

2. Medication Can Decrease Impulsivity in Adults.

The studies of the effects of medication on adults also report decreases in impulsive reactions and emotional reactions such as anger. We have seen this among the adults we work with.

MARSHA *had been diagnosed as hyperactive when she was eight. Her mother's first clue to a problem was the fact that although their back-yard was fenced in, Marsha continually climbed out.*

Throughout her elementary school years, Marsha stayed on medication. When she reached the teen years she seems to calm down, so she was taken off medication.

As an adult, Marsha found it hard not to react quickly to others. She felt impulsive, was often tired and irritable, and found herself get-

ting angry over little things every day. When she finally sought help, she was advised to try medication again.

After taking Ritalin as an adult, Marsha didn't feel the constant stress of trying to inhibit her quick emotional reactions. She felt less "thrown" and more able to handle the little changes or disappointments that occurred. She felt that she got along better with her coworkers and made fewer careless errors, but most of all she didn't make as many rash decisions that led to endless repercussions at home and work.

However, after a "honeymoon period," Marsha found that medication did not change the pattern of how she responded in certain situations. In other words, she was still Marsha. Now, though, with the help of medication, she felt ready to seek additional help to learn how to manage her time, remain calm, and be less reactive and intense about bigger problems.

WHAT MEDICATION CANNOT DO

Although medication can improve attention and reduce distractibility and impulsiveness in some adults, it cannot teach important skills for managing emotions and situations. Medication won't make you someone you are not. It's not designed to do that. Most adults with ADHD have accumulated a number of problems over their lifetime. They may experience anxiety, be depressed, and behave aggressively with others. Medication does not automatically solve all the problems that have grown up as you have.

As with children, medication won't teach adults social skills they never had. Nor will it point you in the correct career path, help you get along with your spouse, or get you to work on time. By the time a person with ADHD reaches adulthood or an untreated adult is diagnosed with ADHD, there may be a number of problems medication cannot improve.

1. Medication Doesn't Improve Self-Esteem or Self-Confidence.

By the time a person with ADHD reaches adulthood, he often has encountered many failures that have lowered his self-esteem. Even a positive response to medication cannot undo the negative self-concept that may inhibit him from trying new ways of succeeding. A fear of failure is one of the greatest handicaps an adult with ADHD has.

2. Medication Doesn't Help the ADHD Adult Find the Right Career or Job.

A particular environment can magnify the characteristics of ADHD, making an adult "more ADHD" than she actually is. In a job that demands close attention to details and concentration on routine tasks, the ADHD adult feels as though he's back in school again. All of his negative traits are intensified. Graham, a master cabinetmaker, said there was no other career he could have succeeded in: "I schedule my own time, enjoy my work, am always moving, and feel success with each piece of furniture I create. I'd be miserable and a failure if I had to sit at a desk, wear a suit, take part in meetings all day."

A bad career match is always a poor choice. It is truly unlikely that medication could make such a significant difference in the life of an ADHD individual that he could become an overnight success in an unsuitable career.

3. Medication Doesn't Organize the Individual.

You probably know it firsthand, and we do, too. Many adults with ADHD have extreme difficulty organizing themselves and their immediate environments. Medication is unlikely to change that. Like the child who has a messy book bag and can't find his homework, the desks of ADHD adults are often piled high with "lost" papers.

Deficits in what has been called the executive function make it difficult for ADHD individuals to plan and sequence activities. As a result, adults with the disorder often have trouble prioritizing activities. They are easily sidetracked and fail to complete important tasks on time, with disastrous results.

Although medication may decrease distractibility and lengthen attention span so the individual is able to get more done at a sitting, it will not turn the typical ADHD adult with years of accumulated mess, missed deadlines, and bad habits into an "Organization Man or Woman."

4. Medication Doesn't Solve Interpersonal Problems.

Many therapists who work with ADHD adults have found that medication doesn't teach them to communicate with others, especially a spouse or significant other. Old habits die hard, and new habits have to be learned. Although medication generally improves impulse control, in emotionally loaded situations involving sensitive issues, people tend to react the way they always have. In such situations, it's even harder for ADHD adults to control their tempers and manage their emotions.

5. Medication Doesn't Solve Psychological or Emotional Problems.

As mentioned previously, additional psychological, behavioral, and emotional problems often coexist with ADHD. Some of these, such as anxiety and depression, may have been caused by the ADHD or could have been primary disorders, existing on their own. Approximately 12 to 30 percent of adults with ADHD have a drug or alcohol problem or some other addiction. A staggering 25 percent exhibit antisocial behaviors or personality disorders. Obviously, medication alone cannot solve such serious problems.

WHAT ELSE YOU CAN DO

Sometimes adults who have not been previously diagnosed as ADHD have become hardened to or learned to live with the traits that trouble them. In this, they're like an adult who doesn't notice the loss of his hearing: he speaks a little louder and misses bits of conversation, but doesn't notice the loss until he finally tries a hearing aid.

Many individuals with ADHD have grown accustomed to their problems. They attribute failure to others or take all the blame on themselves. A diagnosis is like a new lease on life. It offers an explanation for the unexplained and a lead on solutions to the problems that until then have been unsolvable.

GET THE PROPER MEDICAL DIAGNOSIS AND TREATMENT

Many people live all their lives with the traits that characterize ADHD and never know why they can't finish a book, are always late, get angry easily, lose so many jobs, or have difficulty controlling their impulsiveness. One of the most important ways to help yourself is to be certain of the diagnosis. If you elect to try medication, understand what medication can and cannot do, and then do everything you can to improve your situation.

Medication often is erroneously utilized as a diagnostic tool for adults, just as it is with children. And, as with children, your response to medication is not a determinant of the diagnosis. (See chapter 3.)

Here's how to work through the diagnostic process with your physician and other professionals:

- Talk with your physician about the reasons you believe you are ADHD.
- Have a medical exam to eliminate other conditions that may mimic ADHD. See chapter 3 for more detailed information.
- Work through diagnostic procedures for ADHD, including a detailed history and other psychological and psychoeducational tests, to gather information about learning and emotional problems.
- After receiving a diagnosis of ADHD, talk to the appropriate professional people about treatment alternatives, including medication.

Understanding exactly what problems you are dealing with will be an important determiner of the efficacy of medication. For example, is yours a simple case of ADHD or does ADHD exist in combination with other conditions that also require treatment? The information you receive will be crucial in guiding your decision on whether you should try medication and, if so, what type.

Before trying medication, follow the steps outlined in Chapter 4 "What to Try Before You Try Medication." If you still need medication, get the aid of a physician and other professionals who have experience with medications for ADHD, and experience in working with ADHD adults, to monitor your response to medication so that the right dose is determined.

KNOW YOUR ADHD STYLE

ADHD is a very individual matter, and there are many different subtypes of the disorder. What is your pattern? Are you a high-energy type who is always on the go and must be involved in many activities? Are you a daydreamer? Do you find it hard to get yourself going? What types of things do you have trouble concentrating on? Do you become easily overfocused or bogged down in certain types of details so that you are unable to complete the task at hand? Do any coexisting conditions, such as depression or anxiety, complicate your situation? Not all ADHD sufferers are the same. Determine your style or that of your loved one.

EDUCATE YOURSELF ABOUT ADHD

Once an adult knows that ADHD is the cause of many of the problems she has had since childhood, the healing process can begin. Adults emphatically comment that having a diagnosis of ADHD brings about an immense feeling of relief, an immediate lessening of self-criticism, and an increase in self-esteem that had been lowered by years of self-blame. The more you and those you live with understand ADHD, the greater your ability to cope with the disorder and all of the problems it causes.

The education process should begin with the professionals who make the diagnosis and provide treatment. They should share with you a detailed understanding of the ways in which the disorder affects your life and how any accompanying problems affect you. But that is only the beginning. Once you have a diagnosis, you may be amazed at what you learn about yourself. For instance, one of the most poignant stories in Drs. Hallowell and Ratey's book *Driven to Distraction* is the account an ADHD woman shares of her shocking realization of the degree to which ADHD affects every aspect of her life. It is only when she tries medication that she is able to focus enough and become sufficiently less distracted that she has an orgasm for the first time.

Educating yourself is an ongoing process. You should always feel comfortable asking all of your questions. Remember, no question is too basic or too insignificant to ask. You have the right to probe so that you acquire insight about how ADHD affects your daily life and the people in it.

In addition to professional support and firsthand information, there are a number of books on ADHD in adulthood. Or you may find that watching a videotape or listening to a cassette in which individuals with ADHD share their stories better fits your style and interests. A number of excellent resources are listed in the Resource section under "Books, Tapes, and Other Materials."

EDUCATE YOUR PARTNER, OTHER FAMILY MEMBERS, FRIENDS, AND COWORKERS

The literature on ADHD adults is filled with examples of difficulties ADHD adults have in relationships with other adults. Relationships are never simple, but ADHD complicates many of the daily maintenance issues many adults would like to take for granted. Distractibility and impulsive acts can wreak havoc with budgets, bills, and planning. It is very likely the person you live with is just as frustrated as you are by many of the problems associated with the disorder.

Often, ADHD adults are drawn to their opposite type. Your partner is likely to be a great source of help and support for you. However, while your partner may strive to counteract the daily disorganization as well as other problems caused by ADHD, he or she may feel frustrated, puzzled, and angry at having to be responsible for predicaments and difficulties caused by your inattention and impulsiveness. On the other hand, you may feel as though your partner is constantly criticizing you, so that you become bitter and defensive as you protect your already lowered self-esteem.

It's important to educate your significant other about your ADHD symptoms and related problems. Once a sensitive partner understands more about ADHD, it will be easier to once again recognize the good things about you and your relationship that may have been forgotten during the struggle. And as you both better understand how your weaknesses affect daily life, you can work to overcome them with less resentment.

Learning about ADHD often takes on a sense of a "mission" for many ADHD couples. Sometimes the non-ADHD member finds it easier to read and digest information and then share it with the ADHD adult. Others find that by sharing the quest, they learn together. They read or watch videos, attend lectures, and join support groups.

Finally, ADHD affects the entire family. Giving information to other family members, including children, can be very helpful. Since ADHD seems to run in families, the more information all family members have, the more quickly they will recognize problems. Furthermore, as you model the positive ways you overcome the negative characteristics of the disorder, your children and other younger relatives will learn from you. Keep in mind that many of the problems associated with ADHD are a matter of degree. Learning and modeling how to better concentrate, control impulses, and manage social encounters will not go to waste.

There are a number of books in the Resources section that are written for children or other members of your family. Make time to sit down and share what you have learned with them.

GET INDIVIDUAL COUNSELING OR THERAPY

As you know, having ADHD means that you are likely to experience coexisting problems that can damage your self-esteem and affect your daily functioning. Most ADHD adults not only would benefit from but genuinely need some form of counseling or psychotherapy.

Most experts and clinicians in this field believe that therapy is a crucial part of multimodal treatment for ADHD. As Drs. Weiss and Hechtman conclude in the second edition of their classic book *Hyperactive Children Grown Up*, a combination of medication, behavior therapy, and psychotherapy is likely to be the most effective treatment for adult ADHD.

Through psychotherapy, the individual can work to overcome the defensiveness that has become almost an adjunct to an ADHD individual's character. Individual therapy can be an invaluable tool to change long-term patterns that have undermined progress.

Depending on the types of problems you are facing, you should seek therapy from someone who has had experience dealing with the specific problems that trouble you as well as experience dealing with ADHD. If you have an alcohol addiction, for example, you would ideally seek a therapist who is knowledgeable about both ADHD and your particular addiction. The therapist needs to know about any effects the medications used to treat ADHD might have on substance abuse. Don't be afraid to ask potential therapists about their experience in this area.

GET ADDITIONAL HELP AS YOU NEED IT FOR PROBLEMS WITH YOUR RELATIONSHIPS

Working together as a team and acknowledging your need for each other is a major step in coping with the effects of ADHD on your partnership, your life, and your goals. However, there is no added glory to working in isolation. ADHD often leads to serious relationship problems, so don't feel guilty if you and your spouse or family need additional professional help to overcome them.

In fact, having a diagnosis of ADHD may be the permission you need to get help in areas of your life that have bothered you for a long time. You may find that different kinds of help are appropriate at different points in your life.

CHOOSE A THERAPIST WHO UNDERSTANDS
ADHD COUPLES/FAMILIES

In addition to individual counseling, many ADHD adults have relationship problems that often require marital or family therapy. Couples in which one partner is ADHD experience special frustration in a more intense manner. The spouse of an ADHD individual often oscillates between making comments like, "You are never home when you say you'll be," "You didn't think before you . . . ," "You never follow through," or "You don't ever listen to me," and defending the spouse when others make those comments. When one or both partners are ADHD, there are always new challenges for both.

Relationships offer many opportunities for "discussions" about opposing points of view. It is always difficult to deal with the emotionally charged topics every couple has, but ADHD individuals often find it especially difficult to discuss emotional issues. Even in the midst of a conflict about which he feels strongly, an ADHD adult can become distracted or lose his train of thought. Learning to listen to small sound bites and get immediate feedback is an effective way to combat this. Just as the ADHD individual must learn how to break other tasks into manageable segments, communicating requires the same approach.

Many therapists believe that when one or both members of a couple are ADHD, the partnership will be unstable and volatile. Although there is very little controlled research concerning the marital difficulties of ADHD partners, an experienced therapist can help you short-circuit blame and create an environment conducive to solving problems. An effective marital counselor can work with you to develop communication skills that match your style so that old arguments are ended and new solutions are found. In couples therapy, you can work in safe surroundings to learn new ways to improve your lives together so that your love and intimacy are strengthened. What happens in the daytime does affect our nighttime encounters. The effects of medication may be so widespread that the ADHD partner's attention allows him to learn how to relate and respond both verbally and physically in ways that were not possible before.

When looking for help as a couple, search for a therapist who has experience working with ADHD individuals and whose style is active, verbal, and interactive. ADHD adults are unlikely to be successful working with a nondirective, passive therapist. You will benefit from the direct assistance that is offered by a therapist who engages in direct instruction on learning how to communicate safely about emotionally loaded topics.

MATCH YOUR JOB OR CAREER WITH YOUR STYLE

Probably one of the most important factors in feeling successful will be your choice of jobs or career. The right career path makes your life that much easier.

Unfortunately, many adults—whether they have ADHD or not—simply fall into their jobs. If you don't have ADHD, maybe the choice is not as important; you may be one of the lucky people who have many options available. For most ADHD adults, however, there are certain careers that should never be chosen. It is unlikely that someone with ADHD would make a great air traffic controller. Accounting is questionable, since attention to too many details is required. Many adults with ADHD find that paperwork and routine tasks remind them too much of school and homework. They had trouble then and are likely to experience similar problems in routine desk jobs. Sometimes a change of career is in order.

CARY *had struggled for three years working for a major insurance agency. His desk was always piled high, and he could never locate crucial papers when he needed them. Monthly reports were a monthly menace that would have cost him his job if he had not endeared himself to his coworkers. A roamer, he was often away from his desk visiting with others. Luckily, his boss recognized a glimmer of potential there and recommended him to the human resources department. He loved listening to other people's problems and locating resources for them. The demands of his new job changed hourly and daily. He was able to dictate reports, and a secretary kept track of his schedule and deadlines. Along the way Cary had discovered his son was ADHD and realized he too might have the disorder. His second career made sense in the new context.*

If you feel as though you are not reaching your potential in a job or career, you should consider making a change. Seek the guidance of a career counselor or some other professional who is also familiar with

ADHD to help you explore your options. You may decide to take a battery of tests that will offer insight into career options.

FIND THE RIGHT COWORKERS TO SHARE THE JOB

In addition to the right type of job/career, the people you work with can be important factors in your success. Not everyone can have a secretary, but teaming up with others who make you look good is a smart move. Kevin was an extremely talented real estate developer who also had very good "people skills." His hyperactivity fed his enthusiasm and made him quite charismatic. He could work long hours with greater energy and never seem tired. He was also bright enough to realize that his weaknesses were inattention to detail and lack of basic organization skills, but he was clever enough to team up with partners who could manage those functions.

One ADHD adult remarked that finding a "coach" in life was one of the best moves he ever made. An advertising executive who was always going off on creative tangents, he found a friend and coworker to serve as his coach. They met weekly to talk about projects, set priorities, and follow up on commitments. Others in the office probably didn't know that the two men had this special relationship.

JOIN A SUPPORT GROUP

There are various support groups across the country where you will meet people who care about your problems and who are naturally supportive of your efforts to cope. In addition to experiencing the relief of knowing there are others who understand what you're going through, you will meet and learn from the professional advisors who provide up-to-date information and resources. These support groups usually invite monthly speakers to share new information, and often provide lending libraries for their members. Many support groups run special sessions for spouses and family members. You will find information about the network of ADHD support groups in the Resources section under "Organizations and Support Groups That Can Help."

GET HELP BEING ORGANIZED

Face it: Organizational skills are not likely to be your strong point. Rather than struggling and always waiting for tomorrow, work to improve this area today. Try the suggestions listed in Chapter 9, "Routines Medication Does Not Teach." In addition, you may find that an organizational consultant can get you started in this area. Outplacement firms, stores that specialize in organizational materials, career development consultants, and executive trainers may offer valuable advice in this area. Your community college or high school adult education program may also offer a course in this important skill. Individuals with this expertise may come to your home or office and help you set up filing systems, teach you how to use appointment book/calendar systems, and show you other methods for managing your time better. If you are open to suggestions, a spouse, a friend, or a trusted outsider may be able to offer valuable suggestions.

AVOID PUTTING YOURSELF AT RISK

ADHD will always be a double-edged sword, but try to avoid situations in which your ADHD characteristics are likely to cause additional problems or be more noticeable. Know your strengths and weaknesses. For example, if your outgoing nature is about to get you nominated for a position as an officer in an organization which you believe you are particularly unsuited for, and in which you cannot at this time be successful, don't accept the position. Offer your services in another capacity that allows your unique strengths and energy to be put to better use.

Don't get into situations that typically trigger no-win conditions or that generate anger, impulses, and actions that you will later regret. Experiencing guilt for inappropriate behavior is a big issue for ADHD adults.

BUILD YOUR SELF-CONCEPT

Ideally, as you learn and work to overcome the troubling aspects of ADHD, your self-esteem should grow. However, old negative messages are not easy to eliminate. Go on a search-and-destroy mission for old tapes and unexamined critiques that have grown inside your head to monstrous proportions. It's very important to accept and let go of the old baggage. Its weight only impedes your success.

Similarly, avoid creating negative self-fulfilling prophecies based on old messages such as "You're bad. You're stupid. You're never going to amount to anything." Challenge and revise each pessimistic view and replace it with a realistic but positive alternative: "I'm not stupid, I just have an attention deficit disorder." "I'm not bad, I just have difficulty controlling my impulses."

Fill your life with positive experiences that build your self-esteem. Keep a "positive diary" to focus your attention on your positive accomplishments and qualities. Pursue hobbies and activities from which you reap positive feedback as you work to overcome areas of weakness. Getting involved in community activities offers you the opportunity to help others and boost your self-esteem, as well as to put your own problems in better perspective.

HAVE PATIENCE, FORGIVENESS, AND A SENSE OF HUMOR

ADHD individuals often have a hard time forgiving themselves and others. It's not the end of the world when you make a mistake. It's important to laugh and help generate feelings that will make things seem a little lighter. Empathy is the key to dealing with yourself and others.

A FINAL WORD

There is no end of the story for ADHD. Each day, ADHD individuals wake up in the morning and go to bed at night with the special set of characteristics with which they are born. Medication may ease some of the difficulties, but it is up to the individual to learn to manage the cards they were dealt. In addition to the low cards you've been dealt, there are also some aces. The traits that can play havoc with the life of an ADHD individual can also bestow great strength, creativity, enthusiasm, and energy.

As a parent, it is your job to teach your ADHD youngster how to control the traits that cause difficulty so each can become an asset in adulthood. As an adult, you must learn to use your ADHD-related characteristics—both positive and negative—to your advantage. There are many ADHD success stories that prove you can live a happy, successful life. And there are many willing and able people—friends, family members, teachers, physicians, psychologists, and other professionals—who want to help you do that.

RESOURCES

CHILD, ADOLESCENT, AND ADULT

ORGANIZATIONS AND SUPPORT GROUPS THAT CAN HELP

One of the most important things we have stressed in this book is that there is help available for you or your child. The professionals you are working with—your physician, your psychologist, your educational consultant, and others—are available to offer advice, support, and treatment for ADHD. However, there is another set of resources that offer valuable advice, information, and support to parents of children with ADHD and adults who suffer from the disorder.

In the past ten years hundreds of organizations and support groups have sprung up across the country as individuals coping with ADHD have banded together to seek information, solace, support, and encouragement. Organizations have been created to be advocates for you and your child in Washington, D.C., to act as clearinghouses, and to provide a forum for parents to share ideas and gain information. Others act as support groups to offer support and information.

The following organizations and educational resources can offer you help or support in dealing with ADHD and/or learning disabilities.

ADHD ORGANIZATIONS

ADDult Information Exchange Network
c/o Jim Reisinger
P.O. Box 1701
Ann Arbor, MI 48106
(313) 426-1659

The ADDult Information Exchange Network is a nonprofit organization that sponsors an adult ADD conference annually in Ann Arbor, Michigan. The goal is to provide information to adults and adolescents with ADD and professionals who work with these individuals. The network also provides free information and resources.

ADDult Support Network
c/o Mary Jane Johnson, Organizer
2620 Ivy Place
Toledo, OH 43613

The focus of this nonprofit organization is to provide a national network for all adult ADD support groups and adult ADD individuals. It offers a variety of materials including:

1. *ADDult News Newsletter:* A quarterly newsletter with stories, news, and tips that offers an open forum for and by ADD adults. ($15 a year)
2. *INSIDE ADD:* A collection of thoughts and feelings on ADD by an adult who has been there, by Susan Alfutis and edited by Mary Jane Johnson. A seventy-five page spiral book that includes her personal story, journal entries, poems, and artwork. ($16)
3. *ADD—A Lifetime Challenge:* A spiral-bound book edited by Mary Jane Johnson. Each chapter is written by a different ADD adult. ($14.95)
4. *ADDlibs and One Liners:* A sixteen-page booklet that shows the funnier side of life as an ADD person. Written by Susan Alfutis and edited by Mary Jane Johnson. ($6.50)

Attention Deficit Disorder Association
ADDA
P.O. Box 972
Mentor, OH 44061
(800) 487-2282

ADDA is a national organization created to meet the needs of adults with ADD. It serves as a national advocate for ADD-affected individuals in all matters. The founders of ADDA came together in 1988 to work toward common goals, and ADDA is willing to exchange information and offer assistance to help anyone wanting to start a support group. It also holds an annual adult ADD conference.

The Attention Deficit Information Network, Inc.
AD-IN
475 Hillside Avenue
Needham, MA 02194
(617) 455-9895

AD-IN is a nonprofit volunteer organization that offers support and information to families of children and adults with ADD, and to professionals through a network of AD-IN chapters. It was founded in 1988 by several parent support group leaders on the premise of parents' helping parents deal with their children with ADD. The network has parent and adult support group chapters throughout the country.

Children and Adults with Attention Deficit Disorder
CH.A.D.D
National Headquarters
499 NW 70th Avenue, Suite 101
Plantation, FL 33317
(800) 233-4050 (voice mail only) or (305) 587-3700
Fax: (305) 587-3700

CH.A.D.D. is the largest national organization working for people with attention deficit disorders. Ch.A.D.D.'s mission is to help children and adults with ADD achieve success. CH.A.D.D. has local chapters affiliated with it from every state in the United States and sponsors a national conference annually. To find the CH.A.D.D. chapter nearest you, call the national office at (305) 587-3700. This office has an extensive list of chapters that is constantly updated. In addition, the organization offers two regular publications that you can obtain, if you are a member:

1. *The CH.A.D.D.ER Box:* A quarterly, twenty-five-page-plus newsletter that frequently contains articles written by leading researchers and clinicians for adults, children, and families with ADD.
2. *ATTENTION:* A quarterly magazine covering the latest developments in ADD research, diagnosis, and treatments.

Individual dues:	$35 a year
Professional dues:	$65 a year
International dues:	$100 a year (outside United States and Canada)
Organization:	$200 a year
International organization:	$400 a year

Support materials available with membership.

LEARNING DISABILITIES ORGANIZATIONS
Learning Disabilities Association of America
LDA
Jean Peterson, Executive Director
4156 Library Road
Pittsburgh, PA 15234
(412) 341-1515

A national organization with state and local chapters throughout the country. The national headquarters of LDA has available a free packet of information on learning disabilities, including attention deficit disorder. Included in the packet is an extensive resource list of books and pamphlets that are offered for sale. Look in your local telephone book or contact the national office to learn about your local chapter.

National Center for Learning Disabilities
NCLD
381 Park Avenue South, Suite 1420
New York, NY 10016
(212) 545-7510

NCLD is the national center for learning disabilities that was created to promote public awareness and understanding, and to provide national leadership to children and adults with learning disabilities so that they may achieve their potential and enjoy full participation in society.

Membership will entitle you to NCLD publications including *Their World,* quarterly newsletters, periodic news alerts, a packet on learning disabilities, and also invitations to regional and national summits. NCLD also has a free referral service and free literature on a variety of topics, including ADHD.

Individual membership: $35 a year
Institution membership: $50 a year

National Information Center for Children and Youth with Disabilities
NICHY
P.O. Box 1492
Washington, DC 20013-1492

National Network of Learning Disabled Adults
(602) 941-5112

Orton Dyslexia Society
Chester Building
Suite 382
8600 LaSalle Road
Baltimore, MD 21286-2044
(800) ABCD-123 leave message only
(410) 296-0232
Fax: (410) 321-5069

The Orton Dyslexia Society is a scientific and educational organization dedicated to the study and treatment of the specific language disability dyslexia.
There are forty-four local chapters throughout the country, and the national
society can help you find the one nearest you. For $5, the society will send
you a comprehensive basic information packet. Free information is also
available upon request.

EDUCATIONAL RESOURCES
A.D.D. WareHouse
300 NW 70th Avenue, Suite 102
Plantation, FL 33317
(305) 792-8944

An extensive catalog of books, videos, cassettes, and other materials helpful
to those with ADHD and learning disabilities.

ADDendum
c/o CPS
5041 - A Back Lick Road
Annandale, VA 22003
(914) 278-3022

A quarterly newsletter for adults with ADD. Editor: Paul Jaffe; Legal Editor:
Peter Latham, Esq.
($25 per year)

Challenge
c/o Jean Harrison, President
P.O. Box 488
West Newbury, MA 01985
(508) 462-0495

A bimonthly, twelve-page newsletter on attention deficit hyperactivity disorder for children and adults. This newsletter promotes the understanding of

the ADHD child and adult and features a popular section called The Readers' Forum where you can ask specific questions and receive answers from experts in the field. ($25 per year for individuals.)

The Rebus Institute Report
198 Taylor Boulevard, Suite 201
Millbraie, CA 94030
(415) 342-2450

A quarterly newsletter published by the Rebus Institute, a nonprofit research institute devoted to the study and dissemination of information related to adults with learning difficulties and ADD.

STATE ADVOCACY GROUPS
ADD ADVOCACY GROUP
8091 South Ireland Way
Aurora, CO 80016
(303) 690-7548

CH.A.D.D. National State Networking Committee
499 NW 70th Avenue
Suite 101
Plantation, FL 33317
(305) 587-3700

BOOKS, TAPES, AND OTHER MATERIALS

There are many materials available to those who are interested in attention deficit hyperactivity disorder. From surfing bulletin boards on the Internet to watching a video, and from reading books for adults with ADHD and those written for children of all ages, you can find the information you need presented in a style that fits your attention span. Here are some books, tapes, and other materials that we have found to be very informative and helpful in explaining the disorder and its treatment. In addition, we have included a number of books on related subjects that were mentioned in the text of this book.

BOOKS ABOUT ADHD

Barkley, Russell A. *Attention Deficit Hyperactivity Disorder: A Handbook for Diagnosis and Treatment.* New York: The Guilford Press, 1990.

* *The* book on ADHD for professionals. Barkley presents a compendium of research on every aspect of the subject.

Conners, C. Keith. *Feeding the Brain: How Foods Affect Children.* New York and London: Plenum Press, 1989.

* This is the book to read if you are interested in whether allergies or food additives can cause ADHD. Dr. Keith Conners is the author of the well-known Conners Rating Scales.

DuPaul, George J., and Stoner, Gary, with a foreword by Barkley, Russell A. *ADHD in the Schools: Assessment and Intervention Strategies.* New York: The Guilford Press, 1994.

* This book presents an up-to-date understanding of ADHD and strate-

gies for the realities of the school setting. Written for professionals, this is a definitive resource on assessment and intervention in the schools.

Ferber, Richard. *Solve Your Child's Sleep Problems.* New York: A Fireside Book, 1985.
> * An excellent resource to help you determine how much sleep your child needs and to give you suggestions for nighttime problems.

Fowler, Mary Cahill. *Maybe You Know My Kid: A Parent' Guide to Identifying, Understanding and Helping Your Child with Attention Deficit Hyperactivity Disorder.* New York: Birch Lane Press Book, published by Carol Publishing Group, 1990.
> * A mother of an ADHD child sensitively tells the story of her son and how the family dealt with attention deficit disorder.

Garber, Stephen, Ph.D., Garber, Marianne, Ph.D., and Spizman, Robyn Freedman. *Good Behavior.* New York: St. Martin's Press, 1992.
> * We present a practical, easy-to-use guide to solving children's behavior problems, including everything from whining to watching too much television and from boasting to tantrums. The book provides detailed instructions on the effective use of rewards, time-out, overcorrections, and other disciplinary techniques.

If Your Child Is Hyperactive, Inattentive, Impulsive, Distractible . . . Helping the ADD (Attention Deficit Disorder)-Hyperactive Child. New York: Villard, 1990. (Published in trade paperback in 1995 as *Is Your Child Hyperactive? Inattentive? Impulsive? Distractible?: Helping the ADD/Hyperactive Child.*)
> * We present a step-by-step approach for parents to use to teach the ADHD child how to gain self-control, lengthen attention span, and control distractibility and impulsiveness. This straightforward treatment program will help you understand and cope with the challenges of ADHD.

Gordon, Michael. *ADHD/Hyperactivity: A Consumer's Guide: For Parents and Teachers.* DeWitt, NY: GSI Publications, 1991.
> * More than simply a consumer's guide, this is a quick, easy-to-read source for answering basic, practical questions.

My Brother's a World-Class Pain: A Sibling's Guide to ADHD/Hyperactivity. New York: GSI Publications, Inc., 1992.
> * A terrific starting place for a family discussion about ADHD, what it is, and how it affects brothers and sisters of a child with ADHD.

Hallowell, Edward M., M.D., and Ratey, John J., M.D. *Driven to Distraction.* New York: Pantheon Books, 1994.

Answers to Distraction. New York: Pantheon Books, 1994.
* *Driven to Distraction* is an excellent book that addresses how to recognize and cope with attention deficit disorder from childhood through adulthood. *Answers to Distraction* is the authors' response to the most frequently asked questions about attention deficit disorder. We highly recommend both of these books.

Hartmann, Thom, Foreword by Popkin, Michael. *Attention Deficit Disorder: A Different Perception.* Penn Valley, CA: Underwood-Miller, 1993.
* An interesting presentation of a new perception of ADHD. Dr. Hartmann looks at ADHD from a positive viewpoint.

Ingersoll, Barbara D., and Goldstein, Sam. *Attention Deficit Disorder and Learning Disabilities: Reality, Myths and Controversial Treatments.* New York: Doubleday, 1993.
* A comprehensive and helpful resource about attention deficit disorder and learning disabilities, dealing with the causes, symptoms, and diagnoses while also exploring and critiquing possible treatments.

Kendall, Philip C., and Braswell, Lauren. *Cognitive-Behavioral Therapy for Impulsive Children.* New York: The Guilford Press, 1985.
* Although written for professionals, this book presents valuable information about cognitive-behavioral therapy for impulsive children.

Latham, Peter S., and Latham, Pamela H. *Attention Deficit Disorder and the Law.* Washington, D.C.: JKL Communications, 1992.
* An important and helpful resource for every parent who plans to be an advocate for his or her child. Provides a comprehensive understanding of how the law affects ADHD students.

Lee, Christopher, and Jackson, Rosemary. *Faking It: A Look into the Mind of a Creative Learner.* Portsmouth, NH: Boynton/Cook Publishers, 1992.
* One man's story of his struggle and victory in learning to deal with severe learning disabilities. A story of resilience, courage, and the value of support.

Nowicki, Stephen, Jr., and Duke, Marshall. *Helping the Child Who Doesn't Fit In.* Atlanta, GA: Peachtree Publishers, Ltd., 1992.
* Two child psychologists offer parents, teachers, and caretakers a guide to the puzzle of social rejection and its relationship to nonverbal language.

O'Neill, Catherine, illustrated by Goffe, Toni. *Relax.* New York: Child's Play, 1993.

> * A children's book about stress that helps the young child learn how to recognize the symptoms, understand the causes, and find ways to relax body and mind.

Osman, Betty B., in association with Blinder, Henriette. *No One to Play With: The Social Side of Learning Disabilities.* New York: Random House, 1982.

> * This book presents techniques for dealing with the social as well as the academic difficulties learning disabled children face.

Parker, Harvey C. *The ADD Hyperactivity Workbook for Parents, Teachers, and Kids.* Plantation, FL: Specialty Press, 1994.

> * A practical and helpful workbook designed to give information to parents and teachers about ADD and related problems.

Phelan, Thomas W. *All About Attention Deficit Disorder: A Comprehensive Guide.* Glen Ellyn, IL: Child Management Inc, 1993.

> * An easy-to-read guide to attention deficit disorder for parents and teachers, written by an expert on ADHD. Dr. Phelan presents basic advice on the causes, effects, and treatment of ADD.

Quinn, Patricia O., M.D. *ADD and the College Student: A Guide for High School and College Students with Attention Deficit Disorder.* New York: Magination Press, 1994.

> * This book is filled with practical wisdom from both specialists and those who have been there themselves, and offers advice and information to help students with ADHD to effectively navigate the difficult transition to college life.

Turecki, Stanley, M.D., with Wenick, Sarah. *The Emotional Problems of Normal Children: How Parents Can Understand and Help.* New York: Bantam Books, 1994.

> * An excellent resource for understanding the emotional side of your child. Using a step-by-step format, Dr. Turecki shows mothers and fathers how to use their intimate knowledge of the child to understand what's happening—and to intervene effectively.

Umansky, Warren, and Smalley, Barbara Steinberg. *ADD: Helping Your Child: Untying the Knot of Attention Deficit Disorders.* New York: Time Warner Books, 1994.

> * A comprehensive program with practical advice to help children with ADD.

Weiss, Gabrielle, and Hechtman, Lily Trokenberg. *Hyperactive Children Grown Up: ADHD in Children, Adolescents and Adults,* Second Edition. New York: The Guilford Press, 1993.
* The definitive resource on what happens to ADHD children grown up. A summary of the thirty-year longitudinal study of ADHD children at Montreal Children's Hospital.

AUDIO PROGRAMS

Herzfeld, Gerald, and Powell, Robin. *Coping for Kids.* New York: The Center for Applied Research in Education, Inc., 1987.
* A complete stress-control program for students ages eight through eighteen, with audiocassettes and an accompanying book.

VIDEOTAPES

Barkley, Russell A. *ADHD in the Classroom: Strategies for Teachers.* New York: The Guilford Press, 1994.
* An effective video program for teachers about ADHD students in the classroom. Provides valuable information for helping ADHD children at school.

Phelan, Thomas W., and Bloomberg, Jonathan, M.D. *Medication for ADD: Attention Deficit Disorder.* Glen Ellyn, IL: Child Management Inc. (CMI) Products, 1994.
* An up-to-date practical resource for parents, adults, and professionals about medication for ADD.

Phelan, Thomas W. *Adults with Attention Deficit Disorder.* Glen Ellyn, IL: Child Management Inc. (CMI) Products, 1994.
* A videotape for adults with ADD. Real-life experiences shed light on this often confusing disorder and point the way toward successfully dealing with ADD.

AFTERWORD

We continue to learn daily from the children, adolescents, and adults we know and work with. We are interested in your experiences with treatments for ADHD, as well as tips and suggestions you might have discovered that have helped you or your child overcome aspects of this disorder. Often, individuals with an attention deficit disorder hear only the bad news about ADHD. Please send us stories of individuals who have successfully coped with the effects of ADHD.

To share information or to contact us about speeches, workshops, and consulting, we may be reached through:

> The Behavioral Institute of Atlanta
> 5555 Peachtree Dunwoody Road
> Suite 106
> Atlanta, GA 30342
> (404) 256-9325

We can also be reached through e-mail. Our e-mail address is:

> KfYA44A@prodigy.com

If you are interested in receiving a catalog of our materials, please send a stamped, self-addressed envelope to the above address.

REFERENCES

Abikoff, Howard. "Efficacy of Cognitive Training Interventions in Hyperactive Children: A Critical Review." *Clinical Psychology Review* 5 (1985): 479–512.

Abikoff, Howard, et al. "Cognitive Training in Academically Deficient ADDH Boys Receiving Stimulant Medication." *Journal of Abnormal Child Psychology* 16 (1988): 411–432.

Abikoff, Howard, and Gittelman, Rachel. "Hyperactive Children Treated with Stimulants: Is Cognitive Training a Useful Adjunct?" *Archives of General Psychiatry* 42 (1985): 953–961.

Abikoff, Howard, and Gittelman, Rachel. "The Normalizing Effects of Methylphenidate on the Classroom Behavior of ADDH Children." *Journal of Abnormal Child Psychology* 13 (1985): 33–44.

Abramowitz, Ann J., and O'Leary, Susan G. "Behavioral Interventions for the Classroom: Implications for Students with ADHD." *School Psychology Review* 20 (1991): 220–234.

Achenbach, Thomas M., and Edelbrock, Craig S. *Child Behavior Checklist.* Burlington, VT: Achenbach and Edelbrock, 1983.

———. *Child Behavior Checklist—Teacher Report Form.* Burlington, VT: Achenbach and Edelbrock, 1984.

Ayllon, Teodoro, Layman, Dale, and Kandel, Henry. "A Behavioral-Educational Alternative to Drug Control of Hyperactive Children." *Journal of Applied Behavior Analysis* 8 (1975): 137–146.

Ayres, Jean. *Sensory Integration and Learning Disorders.* Los Angeles: Western Psychological Services, 1973.

Baer, Ruth A., and Nietzel, Michael T. "Cognitive and Behavioral Treatment of Impulsivity in Children: A Meta-Analytic Review of the Outcome Literature." *Journal of Clinical Child Psychology* 20 (1991): 400–412.

Barkley, Russell A. *Attention Deficit Hyperactivity Disorder: A Handbook for Diagnosis and Treatment.* New York: The Guilford Press, 1990.

Barrickman, Les, et al. "Treatment of ADHD with Fluoxetine: A Preliminary Trial." *Journal of American Academy of Child and Adolescent Psychiatry* 30 (1991): 762–767.

Bass, Alison. "More Mass. Pupils Get Ritalin, and Doubts Rise." *The Boston Globe:* A:1.

Benson, Herbert. *The Relaxation Response.* New York: William Morrow, 1975.

Bloomquist, Michael L., August, Gerald J., and Ostrander, Rick. "Effects of a School-Based Cognitive-Behavioral Intervention for ADHD Children." *Journal of Abnormal Psychology* 19 (1991): 591–605.

Bornstein, P., and Quevillon, R. P. "The Effects of a Self-Instructional Package on Overactive Preschool Boys." *Journal of Applied Behavior Analysis* 9 (1976): 179–188.

Braswell, Lauren. "Cognitive-Behavioral Groups for Children Manifesting ADHD and Other Disruptive Behavior Disorders." *Special Services in the Schools* 8 (1993): 91–117.

Brown, Ronald T., et al. "Methylphenidate and Cognitive Therapy with ADD Children: A Methodological Reconsideration." *Journal of Abnormal Child Psychology* 14 (1986): 481–497.

Buhrmester, Duane, et al. "Prosocial Behavior in Hyperactive Boys: Effects of Stimulant Medication and Comparison with Normal Boys." *Journal of Abnormal Child Psychology* 20 (1992): 103–121.

Carlson, Caryn L., and Thomeer, Marcus L. "Effects of Ritalin on Arithmetic Tasks." In Greenhill, Laurence L., M.D., and Osman, Betty B., Ph.D., Editors. *Ritalin Theory and Patient Management.* New York: Mary Ann Liebert, Inc., Publishers, 1991: 195–202.

Comings, David E., M.D., et al. "The Clonidine Patch and Behavior Problems." *Journal of the American Academy of Adolescent Psychiatry* 29 (1990): 667–668.

Conners, C. Keith. "The Computerized Continuous Performance Test. *Psychopharmacology Bulletin* 21 (1985): 891–892.

———. *Conners Parent Rating Scale—Revised.* _____: North Tonawanda, NY: Multi-Health Systems, Inc., 1989.

———. *Conners Teacher Rating Scale—Revised.* _____: North Tonawanda, NY: Multi-Health Systems, Inc., 1989.

———. *Feeding the Brain: How Foods Affect Children.* New York: Plenum Press, 1989.

———. "A Teacher Rating Scale for Use in Drug Studies with Children." *American Journal of Psychiatry* 126 (1969) : 884–888.

Conners, C. Keith, and Wells, Karen D. *Hyperkinetic Children.* Beverly Hills: Sage Publications, 1986.

Copeland, Edna D., Ph.D., and Copps, Stephen C., M.D. *Medications for Atten-*

tion Disorders (ADHD/ADD) and Related Medical Problems. Plantation, FL: Specialty Press, Inc., 1995.

Copeland, Linda, M.D., et al. "Pediatricians' Reported Practices in the Assessment and Treatment of Attention Deficit Disorder." *Developmental and Behavioral Pediatrics* 8 (1987): 191–196.

Crook, William G. *The Yeast Connection: A Medical Breakthrough.* Jackson, TN: Professional Books, 1986.

Diagnostic Criteria from DSM-IV. Washington, D.C.: The American Psychiatric Association, 1994.

Diener, Robert M. "Toxocology of Ritalin." In Greenhill, Laurence L., M.D., and Osman, Betty B., Ph.D., Editors. *Ritalin Theory and Patient Management.* New York: Mary Ann Liebert, Inc., Publishers, 1991: 195–202.

Douglas, Virginia. "Stop, Look, and Listen: The Problem of Sustained Attention and Impulse Control in Hyperactive and Normal Children." *Canadian Journal of Behavioral Science* 4 (1972): 159–182.

"Drugs for Psychiatric Disorders." *The Medical Letter* 36 (October 14, 1994): 89–96.

DuPaul, George J., and Barkley, Russell A. "Behavior Contributions to Pharmacotherapy: The Utility of Behavioral Methodology in Medication Treatment of Children with Attention Deficit Hyperactivity Disorder." *Behavior Therapy* 24 (1993): 467–465.

DuPaul, George J., Barkley, Russell A., and McMurray, Mary B. "Therapeutic Effects of Medication on ADHD: Implications for School Psychologists." *School Psychology Review* 20 (1991): 203–219.

DuPaul, George J., Guevremont, David C., and Barkley, Russell A. "Behavior Treatment of Attention Deficit Hyperactivity Disorder in the Classroom: The Use of the Attention Training System." *Journal of Abnormal Child Psychology* 20 (1992): 213–232.

DuPaul, George J., and Hennington, Patricia N. "Peer Tutoring Effects on the Classroom Performance of Children with Attention Deficit Hyperactivity Disorder." *School Psychology Review* 22 (1993): 134–143.

DuPaul, George J., Ph.D., and Stoner, Gary, Ph.D. *ADHD in the Schools.* New York: The Guilford Press, 1994.

Elia, Josephine, and Rapoport, Judith L., "Ritalin versus Dextroamphetamine in ADHD: Both Should Be Tried." In Greenhill, Laurence L., M.D., and Osman, Betty B., Ph.D., Editors. *Ritalin Theory and Patient Management.* New York: Mary Ann Liebert, Inc., Publishers, 1991: 69–74.

Evans, Steven W., and Pelham, William E. "Psychostimulant Effects on Academic and Behavioral Measures for ADHD Junior High School Students in a Lecture Format Classroom." *Journal of Abnormal Child Psychology* 19 (1991): 537–551.

Famularo, Richard, M.D., and Fenton, Terence, Ed.D. "The Effect of Methylphenidate on School Grades in Children with Attention Deficit

Disorder without Hyperactivity: A Preliminary Report." *Journal of Clinical Psychiatry* 48 (1987): 112–114.

Feingold, Benjamin F. *Why Your Child Is Hyperactive.* New York: Random House, 1975.

Feldman, Heidi, Levine, Melvine D., and Fenton, Terence. "Estimating Personal Performance: A Problem for Children with School Dysfunction." *Journal of Developmental and Behavioral Pediatrics* 7 (1986): 281–287.

Fiore, Thomas A., Becker, Elizabeth A., and Nero, Rebecca C. "Educational Interventions for Students with Attention Deficit Disorder." *Exceptional Children* 60 (1993): 163–173.

Fine, Stuart, M.B., and Johnston, Charlotte, Ph.D., "Drug and Placebo Side Effects in Methylphenidate-Placebo Trial for Attention Deficit Hyperactivity Disorder." *Child Psychiatry and Human Development* 24 (1993): 25–30.

Foster, Catherine. "Controversy Over Using Drugs to Control Children's Behavior." *Christian Science Monitor,* January 28, 1988: 19.

Gadow, Kenneth D., and Nolan, Edith. "Practical Considerations in Conducting School-Based Medication Evaluations in Children with Hyperactivity." *Journal of Emotional and Behavioral Disorders.* 1 (1993): 118–121.

Golden, Gerald S., M.D., "Commentary: The Myth of Attention Deficit-Hyperactivity Disorder." *Journal of Child Neurology* 7 (1992): 446–461.

Goldstein, Sam, and Ingersoll, Barbara. "Controversial Treatments for Children with Attention Deficit Disorder." *CH.A.D.D.ER Box,* Fall/Winter 1992: 19–22.

Gomez, Karen M., and Cole, Christine L. "Attention Deficit Hyperactivity Disorder: A Review of Treatment Alternatives." *Elementary School Guidance and Counseling* 26 (1991): 106–114.

Gordon, M. *The Gordon Diagnostic System.* Dewitt, NY: Clinical Diagnostic Systems, 1983.

Gordon, Michael, et al. "Nonmedical Treatment of ADHD/Hyperactivity: The Attention Training System." *Journal of School Psychology* 29 (1991): 151–159.

Gordy, Peter. "Think Twice Before Drugging Kids." *The Atlanta Journal and Constitution,* February 5, 1995: B:7.

Greenhill, Laurence L., M.D., and Osman, Betty B., Ph.D., Editors. *Ritalin Theory and Patient Management.* New York: Mary Ann Liebert, Inc., Publishers, 1991.

Hall, Cathy W., and Kataria, Sudesh. "Effects of Two Treatment Techniques on Delay and Vigilance Tasks with Attention Deficit Hyperactive Disorder (ADHD) Children." *Journal of Psychology* 126 (1992): 17–25.

Hallowell, Edward M., M.D., and Ratey, John J., M.D., *Driven to Distraction.* New York: Pantheon Books, 1994.

Hamlett, Kim W., Pellegrini, David S., and Conners, C. Keith. "An Investigation of Executive Processes in the Problem-Solving of Attention Deficit Disorder-Hyperactive Children." *Journal of Pediatric Psychology* 12 (1987): 227–239.

Henker, Barbara, et al. "Does Stimulant Medication Improve the Peer Status of Hyperactive Children?" *Journal of Consulting and Clinical Psychology* 57 (1989): 545–549.

Hinshaw, Stephen P., et al. "Aggressive, Prosocial, and Nonsocial Behavior in Hyperactive Boys: Dose Effects of Methylphenidate in Naturalistic Settings." *Journal of Consulting and Clinical Psychology* 52 (1989): 636–643.

Horn, Wade F., Chatoor, Irene, and Conners, C. Keith. "Additive Effects of Dexedrine and Self-Control Training: A Multiple Assessment." *Behavior Modification* 7 (1983): 383–402.

Hunt, Robert D., Lau, Serena, and Ryu, Jeff. "Alternative Therapies for ADHD." In Greenhill, Laurence L., M.D., and Osman, Betty B., Ph.D., Editors. *Ritalin Theory and Patient Management.* New York: Mary Ann Liebert, Inc., Publishers, 1991: 75–95.

Ingersoll, Barbara D., Ph.D., and Goldstein, Sam, Ph.D. *Attention Deficit Disorder and Learning Disabilities: Reality, Myths and Controversial Treatments.* New York: Doubleday, 1993.

Jackson, Nancy F., Jackson, Donald A., and Monroe, Cathy. *Getting Along with Others: Teaching Social Effectiveness to Children.* Champaign, IL: Research Press, 1983.

Jacobson, Edmund, Ph.D. *You Must Relax.* New York: McGraw-Hill, 1934.

Janzen, Troy, et al. "Differences in Baseline EEG Measures for ADD and Normally Achieving Preadolescent Males." *Biofeedback and Self-Regulation* 20 (1995): 65–82.

Kelly, Jeffrey A. "Group Social Skills Training." *The Behavior Therapist* 8 (1985): 93–95.

Kendall, Philip C. "Cognitive-Behavioral Therapies with Youth: Guiding Theory, Current Status, and Emerging Developments." *Journal of Consulting and Clinical Psychology* 61 (1993): 235–247.

Kendall, Philip C., and Braswell, Lauren. *Cognitive-Behavioral Therapy for Impulsive Children.* New York: The Guilford Press, 1985.

Laccetti, Susan. "Parent Sues Over Use of Ritalin to Treat Pupils." November 10, 1987: A:33.

———. "60% Increase in Use of Ritalin Spurs Call for National Review." *Atlanta Journal and Constitution,* April 13, 1987: A:1.

Latham, Peter, S., and Latham, Patricia H. *Attention Deficit Disorder and the Law.* Washington, D.C. : JKL Communications, 1992.

Leary, Warren E. "Blunder Limits Supply of Crucial Drug." *The New York Times*, November 14, 1993: I:20.

Lee, Christopher, and Jackson, Rosemary F. *Faking It: A Look into the Mind of a Creative Learner*. Portsmouth, NH: Boynton/Cook Publishers, 1992.

Leff, Lisa. "Md. [Maryland] Seeks Way to Put a Lid on Prescription Drug Abuse." *The Washington Post*, November 26, 1989: D:1.

Levinson, Harold N., *Total Concentration: How to Understand Attention Deficit Disorder, Maximize Your Mental Energy, and Reach Your Full Potential*. New York: M. Evans, 1992.

Levy, Doug. "Tight Supply of Hyperactivity Drug." *USA Today*, November 10, 1993: D:5.

Levy, Florence. "CNS Stimulant Controversies." *Australian and New Zealand Journal of Psychiatry* 23 (1989): 497–502.

Lubar, Joel F., et al. "Evaluation of the Effectiveness of EEG Neurofeedback Training for ADHD in a Clinical Setting as Measured by Changes in T.O.V.A. Scores, Behavioral Ratings, and WISC-R Performance." *Biofeedback and Self-Regulation* 20 (1995): 83–99.

McBurnett, Keith, Lahey, Benjamin B., and Swanson, James M. "Ritalin Treatment in Attention Deficit Disorder without Hyperactivity." In Greenhill, Laurence L., M.D., and Osman, Betty B., Ph.D., Editors. *Ritalin Theory and Patient Management*. New York: Mary Ann Liebert, Inc., Publishers, 1991: 257–263.

McKinney, James D., Montague, Marjorie, and Hocutt, Anne M. "Educational Assessment of Students with Attention Deficit Disorder." *Exceptional Children* 60 (1993): 125–131.

Macklin, Gayle L. "No One Wants to Play With Me." *Academic Therapy* 22 (1987): 477–484.

Mannuzza, Salvatore, et al. "Adult Outcome of Hyperactive Boys." *Archives of General Psychiatry* 50 (1993): 565–576.

Mattes, J.A., and Gittelman, R. "Growth of Hyperactive Children on Maintenance Regimen of Methylphenidate." *Archives of General Psychiatry* 40 (1983): 317–321.

Meichenbaum, D., and Goodman, J. "Training Impulsive Children to Talk to Themselves: A Means of Developing Self-Control." *Journal of Abnormal Psychology* 72 (1971): 240–249.

Merewood, Anne. "Seeing Clearly Now." *Child.* October 1992: 58–63.

Milich, Richard, and Pelham, William E. "Effects of Sugar Ingestion on the Classroom and Playgroup Behavior of Attention Deficit Disordered Boys." *Journal of Consulting and Clinical Psychology* 54 (1986): 714–718.

Millenson, Michael L. "Questions Raised on Use of Hyperactivity Drugs." *The Chicago Tribune*, October 21, 1988: I:2.

Neilans, T. H., and Israel, A. C. "Towards Maintenance and Generalization of Behavior Change: Teaching Children Self-Instructional Skills." *Cognitive Therapy and Research* 5 (1981): 189–196.

Osman, Betty B. "Coordinating Care in the Prescription and Use of Methylphenidate with Children." In Greenhill, Laurence L., M.D., and Osman, Betty B., Ph.D., Editors. *Ritalin Theory and Patient Management.* New York: Mary Ann Liebert, Inc., Publishers, 1991: 119–129.

Pelham, William E., and Milich, Richard. "Individual Differences in Response to Ritalin in Classwork and Social Behavior." In Greenhill, Laurence L., M.D., and Osman, Betty B., Ph.D., Editors. *Ritalin Theory and Patient Management.* New York: Mary Ann Liebert, Inc., Publishers, 1991: 203–219.

Peloquin, Lori J., and Klorman, Rafael. "Effects of Methylphenidate on Normal Children's Mood, Event-Related Potentials, and Performance in Memory Scanning and Vigilance." *Journal of Abnormal Psychology* 95 (1986): 88–98.

Perl, Rebecca. "Atlanta Leads South in Ritalin Prescriptions." *The Atlanta Journal and Constitution,* November 8, 1992: A:1.

———. "Overdoses Raise Questions about Alternative Drug." *The Atlanta Journal and Constitution,* November 8, 1992: D:6.

———. "Overdosing on Ritalin?" *The Atlanta Journal and Constitution,* November 8, 1992: D:1.

Rapoport, Judith L., et al. "Dextroamphetamine: Its Cognitive and Behavioral Effects in Normal and Hyperactive Boys and Normal Men." *Archives of General Psychiatry* 37 (1980): 933–943.

Rapport, Mark D. "Hyperactivity and Frustration: The Influence of Control Over and Size of Rewards in Delaying Gratification." *Journal of Abnormal Child Psychology* 14 (1986): 191–204.

Rapport, Mark D., et al. "Attention Deficit Disorder with Hyperactivity and Methylphenidate: The Effects of Dose and Mastery Level on Children's Learning Performance." *Journal of Abnormal Child Psychology* 17 (1989): 669–689.

Rapport, Mark D., et al. "Attention Deficit Disorder and Methylphenidate: A Multilevel Analysis of Dose-Response Effects and Children's Impulsivity Across Settings." *Journal of the American Academy of Child and Adolescent Psychiatry* 27 (1988): 60–69.

Rapport, Mark D., et al. "Methylphenidate in Hyperactive Children: Differential Effects of Dose on Academic, Learning, and Social Behavior." *Journal of Abnormal Child Psychology* 13 (1985): 227–244.

Rapport, Mark D., Murphy, H. Allen, and Bailey, Jon S. "The Effects of a Response Cost Treatment Tactic on Hyperactive Children." *Journal of School Psychology* 18 (1980): 98–111.

————. "Ritalin vs. Response Cost in the Control of Hyperactive Children: A Within-Subject Comparison." *Journal of Applied Behavior Analysis* 15 (1982): 205–216.

Ratey, John J., et al. "Unrecognized Attention-Deficit Hyperactivity Disorder in Adults Presenting for Outpatient Psychotherapy." *Journal of Child and Adolescent Psychopharmacology* 2 (1992): 267–275.

Redman, Christine A., and Zametkin, Alan J. "Ritalin and Brain Metabolism." In Greenhill, Laurence L., M.D., and Osman, Betty B., Ph.D., Editors. *Ritalin Theory and Patient Management.* New York: Mary Ann Liebert, Inc., Publishers, 1991: 195–202.

Rochell, Anne. "Ritalin Shortage Putting Users on Edge." *The Atlanta Journal and Constitution,* November 4, 1993: G:1.

Sappell, Joel, and Welkos, Robert W. "Suits, Protests Fuel a Campaign Against Psychiatry." *Los Angeles Times,* June 29, 1990: A:48.

Scarnati, D.O., Richard. "An Outline of Hazardous Side Effects of Ritalin." *The International Journal of the Addictions* 21 (1986): 837–841.

Schiff, Matthew M., and Cavaiola, Alan A. "Teenage Chemical Dependence and the Prevalence of Psychiatric Disorders: Issues for Prevention." *Journal of Adolescent Chemical Dependency* 2 (1990): 35–46.

Schmidt, William E. "Sales of Drug Are Soaring for Treatment of Hyperactivity." *The New York Times,* May 5 1987: C:3.

Seidel, William T., and Joschko, Michael. "Evidence of Difficulties in Sustained Attention in Children with ADDH." *Journal of Abnormal Child Psychology* 18 (1990): 217–229.

Sergeant, Joseph A., and Van-der-Meere, Jaap. "What Happens After a Hyperactive Child Commits an Error" *Psychiatry Research* 24 (1988): 157–164.

Shaywitz, Sally E., and Shaywitz, Bennett A. "Attention Deficit Disorder: Diagnosis and Role of Ritalin in Management." In Greenhill, Laurence L., M.D., and Osman, Betty B., Ph.D., Editors. *Ritalin Theory and Patient Management.* New York: Mary Ann Liebert, Inc., Publishers, 1991.

Sherman, Miriam, and Hertzig, Margaret. "Prescribing Practices of Ritalin: The Suffolk County, New York Study." In Greenhill, Laurence L., M.D., and Osman, Betty B., Ph.D., Editors. *Ritalin Theory and Patient Management.* New York: Mary Ann Liebert, Inc., Publishers, 1991: 187–193.

Shulman, Victor, M.D. "Medical Management of Attention Deficit Hyperactivity Disorder." CH.A.D.D.ER Box Fall/Winter (1987): 6–7.

Simeon, Jovan G., M.D., and Wiggins, Doreen M. "Pharmacotherapy of Attention-Deficit Hyperactivity Disorder." *Canadian Journal of Psychiatry* 38 (1993): 443–448.

Solanto, Mary V. "Dosage Effects of Ritalin on Cognition." In Greenhill, Laurence L., M.D., and Osman, Betty B., Ph.D., Editors. *Ritalin Theory and Patient Management.* New York: Mary Ann Liebert, Inc., Publishers, 1991: 233–245.

Stroebel, Charles F. *The Quieting Response.* Manual and Audio Cassette Program. New York: BMA Publications, 1978.

"Sugar Highs." *The Atlanta Journal and Constitution,* March 15, 1995: G:3.

Ullmann, Rina K., Ph.D., et al. *ADD-H Comprehensive Teacher Rating Scale.* Institute for Child Behavior and Development, Champaign, IL: 1984.

Vyse, Stuart A., and Rapport, Mark D. "The Effects of Methylphenidate on Learning in Children with ADDH: The Stimulus Equivalence Paradigm." *Journal of Consulting and Clinical Psychology* 57 (1989): 425–435.

Walker, Chyril J., and Clement, Paul W. "Treating Inattentive, Impulsive, Hyperactive Children with Self-Modeling and Stress Inoculation Training." *Child and Family Behavior Therapy* 14 (1992): 75–85.

Ward, Mark F., Ph.D., Wender, Paul H., M.D., and Reimherr, Fred W., M.D. "The Wender Utah Rating Scale: An Aid in the Retrospective Diagnosis of Childhood Attention Deficit Hyperactivity Disorder." *American Journal of Psychiatry* 150 (1993): 885–891.

Weiss, Gabrielle, and Hechtman, Lily Trokenberg. *Hyperactive Children Grown Up: ADHD in Children, Adolescents and Adults,* Second Edition. New York: The Guilford Press, 1993.

Weiss, Lynn. *Attention Deficit Disorder in Adults.* Dallas: Taylor Publishing Company, 1992.

Wender, Esther H., M. D., and Solanto, Mary V., Ph. D. "Effects of Sugar on Aggressive and Inattentive Behavior in Children with Attention Deficit Disorder with Hyperactivity and Normal Children." Pediatrics 88 (1991): 960–966.

Wender, Paul, Wood, D. R., and Reimherr, F. W. "Pharmacological Treatment of Attention Deficit Disorder, Residual Type." *Psychopharmacology Bulletin* 21 (1985): 222–231.

Whalen, Carol K., et al. "Messages of Medication: Effects of Actual versus Informed Medication Status on Hyperactive Boys' Expectancies and Self-Evaluation." *Journal of Consulting and Clinical Psychology* 59 (1991): 602–606.

Whalen, Carol K., and Henker, Barbara. "Therapies for Hyperactive Children: Comparisons, Combinations and Compromises." *Journal of Consulting and Clinical Psychology* 59 (1991): 127–137.

Whalen, Carol K., Henker, Barbara, and Granger, Douglas A. "Social Judgment Processes in Hyperactive Boys: Effects of Methylphenidate and Comparisons with Normal Peers." *Journal of Abnormal Child Psychology* 18 (1990): 297–316.

Whalen, Carol K., Henker, Barbara, and Hinshaw, Stephen P. "Cognitive-Behavioral Therapies for Hyperactive Children: Premises, Problems and Prospects." *Journal of Abnormal Child Psychology* 13 (1985): 391–410.

Williams, Linda. "Parents and Doctors Fear Growing Misuse of Drug Used to Treat Hyperactive Kids." *The Wall Street Journal,* January 15, 1988: 21.

Woltersdorf, Mitchel A. "Videotape Self-Modeling in the Treatment of Attention-Deficit Hyperactivity Disorder." *Child and Family Behavior Therapy* 14 (1992): 53–73.

Wood, D.R., et al. "Diagnosis and Treatment of Minimal Brain Dysfunction in Adults." *Archives of General Psychiatry* 33 (1976): 1453–1460.

Wright, Jeanne. "Tuning In to Concentrate." *Los Angeles Times,* October 4, 1992: E:9.

Yancey, Wanda R. "Gwinnett Mom Asks $50 Million in Suit on Son's Ritalin Use." *The Atlanta Journal and Constitution,* January 19, 1989: C:2.

Zentall, Sydney S. "Research on the Educational Implications of Attention Deficit Hyperactivity Disorder." *Exceptional Children* 60 (1993): 143–153.

INDEX

educational resources, 225–26
EEG (brain wave tests), 39
Elia, Josephine, 89, 93
Emory University, 72
Emotional Problems of Normal Children, The (Turecki), 230
emotional/psychological problems, 39–43
  anxiety, 13–14, 39–41, 200–1, 208
  behavior disorders, 42
  dealing with emotions, 127–28, 161
  depression, 41–42, 200–1, 208
  and medication, 208
  thought disorders, 42–43, 201
environmental modifications
  for adults, 78–81
  for children and adolescents, 58–65, 112–13
  at home, 64–65
  at school, 58–64, 112–13
  at work, 78–81, 214–17
environmental scan, 171
executive functioning, 159, 207
expressive language problems, 110
eye contact
  in greetings, 133
  making, 134
eye problems, 33–35, 110

Faking It (Lee and Jackson), 44, 229
family members, educating about ADHD, 100–1, 210–11
family therapy, 213–14
Famularo, Richard, 107
feedback
  biofeedback/neurofeedback, 194
  home-school system, 74–76, 114
  on medication, 88, 101–2
  on social skills, 136
  from teachers, 61–62, 74–76, 88, 101–2, 113, 114
Feeding the Brain (Conners), 188, 227
Feingold, Benjamin, 38, 188
Feingold diet, 38, 188–89
Fenton, Terence, 107
Ferber, Richard, 228
Fidgety Phil, 10–11, see also attention deficit hyperactivity disorder (ADHD)
"fight or flight" response, 180
file drawers, 168

food additives, 38, 188–89
Food and Drug Administration, U.S. (FDA), 10, 104
forgetfulness, and medication, 162
forgiveness, 217
Foundation Health, 30
Fowler, Mary Cahill, 228
friends, educating about ADHD, 100–1, 210–11

Gadow, Kenneth, 98
Garber, Marianne, 228
Garber, Stephen, 228
Georgia State University, 73, 114
Gittelman, Rachel, 91, 106
glucose tolerance tests, 37
Goldman, Jane, 189–90
Goldstein, Sam, 229
Good Behavior (Garber, Garber, and Spizman), 170, 228
Goodman, J., 146
Gordon, Michael, 73, 100, 228
Gordon Diagnostic System, 50, 177
grades, impact of medication on, 107
grandparents, explaining ADHD to, 100–1
Greenberg, Lawrence, 50
group dynamics, 126–27
growth, stunted, 4, 14–17, 91

habits
  developing, 165
  positive reinforcement for, 166
Hallowell, Edward M., 210, 229
hallucinations, 42, 43
hallucinogens, 18
haloperidol, 97
handwriting, 20, 160
happiness, and medication, 130
Hartmann, Thom, 229
Harvard Medical School, 107
Harvard University, 183
headaches, and stimulants, 90
hearing difficulties, 35
Hechtman, Lily Trokenberg, 76, 98, 105, 146, 200, 212, 231
height, and ADHD medication, 4, 14–17, 91
Helping the Child Who Doesn't Fit In (Nowicki and Duke), 229
Henker, Barbara, 29–30

ABOUT THE AUTHORS

STEPHEN W. GARBER, PH.D., is one of the country's leading parenting experts and is the director of the Behavioral Institute in Atlanta. MARIANNE DANIELS GARBER, PH.D., is an educational consultant at the Behavioral Institute and is an adviser to parents, teachers, and other specialists. ROBYN FREEDMAN SPIZMAN has published sixty books and numerous articles on enhancing children's learning. They are the authors of *Is Your Child Hyperactive? Inattentive? Impulsive? Distractible? Helping the ADD/ Hyperactive Child; Good Behavior;* and *Monsters Under the Bed.* They live in Atlanta.

T